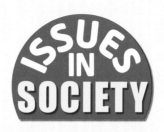

How Harmful Are Performance-Enhancing Drugs?

John Allen

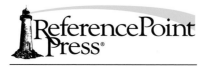

ReferencePoint Press®

San Diego, CA

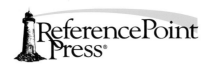

© 2017 ReferencePoint Press, Inc.
Printed in the United States

For more information, contact:
ReferencePoint Press, Inc.
PO Box 27779
San Diego, CA 92198
www.ReferencePointPress.com

LIBRARY OF CONGRESS CATALOGING-IN-PUBLICATION DATA

Names: Allen, John, 1957- author.
Title: How harmful are performance-enhancing drugs? / by John Allen.
Description: San Diego, CA : ReferencePoint Press, Inc., 2017. | Series: Issues in society | Audience: Grade 9 to 12. | Includes bibliographical references and index.
Identifiers: LCCN 2016004056 (print) | LCCN 2016005947 (ebook) | ISBN 9781682820766 (hardback) | ISBN 9781682820773 (eBook)
Subjects: LCSH: Doping in sports.
Classification: LCC RC1230 .A42 2017 (print) | LCC RC1230 (ebook) | DDC 362.29/088796--dc23
LC record available at http://lccn.loc.gov/2016004056

CONTENTS

A Secret Doping Program

In the fiercely competitive world of international sports, nations go to great lengths to get the slightest edge. On November 9, 2015, the World Anti-Doping Agency (WADA) released a report accusing Russia of engaging in state-sponsored doping to improve its athletes' performance. The report alleged that the secret doping program went back five years and involved Russian officials, physicians, coaches, and athletes. The program aimed to give Russian athletes an illicit advantage in international competitions, including the Olympics, by providing them with banned performance-enhancing drugs, or PEDs.

Based on the report's findings, WADA recommended that Russia's track and field team be banned from the 2016 Olympics in Rio de Janeiro. Although Russian sports minister Vitaly Mutko was quick to deny the allegations, WADA officials insisted the evidence was overwhelming. "It's worse than we thought," said Dick Pound, head of the three-person commission that produced the report. "We found coverups, we found destruction of samples, we found payments of money in order to conceal doping tests."[1] Athletes who refused to go along with the doping scheme were threatened with expulsion from their team—and some feared even more drastic consequences. One Russian athlete told the WADA commission that anyone with doubts about the doping program would think, "Leave it, otherwise you might accidentally get in a car accident."[2]

A Long Line of Scandals

Sports fans worldwide have grown accustomed to doping scandals. Perhaps the most high-profile offender is Lance Armstrong, the American cyclist. After years of denying any wrongdoing, Armstrong finally admitted in 2013 that he used banned substances to win his record-breaking seven titles in the Tour de France, the world's most prestigious—and grueling—bicycle race. Armstrong's admission only added to the public's understandable cynicism about the use of performance-enhancing drugs in sports. In May 2015 the entire US men's sprint relay team was stripped of its silver medal in the 2012 London Olympics due to Tyson Gay's doping. Major League Baseball (MLB) suspended New York Yankees infielder Alex Rodriguez for the entire 2014 season for PED use. Milwaukee Brewers slugger Ryan Braun also was caught doping and sat out half the 2013 season. The 2002 BALCO (Bay Area Laboratory Co-Operative) scandal implicated elite athletes in several sports, including baseball's all-time home run champion Barry Bonds, track-and-field gold medal winner Marion Jones, and National Football League (NFL) all-pro linebacker Bill Romanowski. The 2004 Athens Olympics, probably the worst in history for PED violations, saw 26 doping cases come to light, including implicating six medalists, two of them gold medal winners. Retroactive tests

> "[The use of PEDs by Russian athletes is] worse than we thought. We found coverups, we found destruction of samples, we found payments of money in order to conceal doping tests."[1]
>
> —Dick Pound, head of the three-person WADA commission.

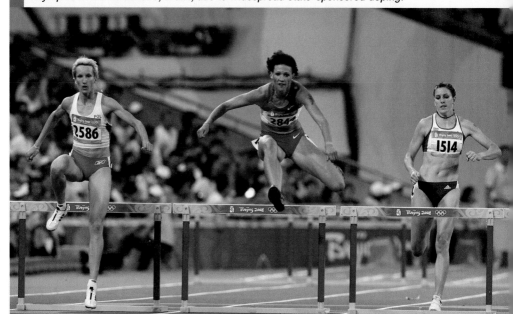

Russian athlete Yekaterina Bikert (center) competes in the 400m hurdles against Poland's Anna Jesien (left) and the Czech Republic's Zuzana Hejnova (right) during the 2008 Olympics in Beijing, China. In November 2015, the World Anti-Doping Agency recommended that Russia's track and field team be banned from the 2016 Olympics in Rio de Janeiro, Brazil, due to widespread state-sponsored doping.

have raised those totals to eleven medalists and three winners of gold. It often seems as if no sport is immune. Even the Professional Golfers Association Tour has suspended players for using banned substances.

Polls show that sports fans tend to have mixed feelings about PED use. Fans suspect that drug use in sports is more widespread than is generally acknowledged, and they claim to dislike the influence of drugs in sports. In one 2013 poll of baseball fans, 60 percent of those surveyed said it matters to them a lot if players use steroids or other PEDs. Only 9 percent said PED use was not an important issue. Yet despite several scandals over steroid use, MLB continues to enjoy high attendance figures and strong television ratings. When Ryan Braun returned to the Brewers' lineup after his suspension for steroid use, Milwaukee fans gave him a standing ovation. As NBC Sports reporter Craig Calcaterra observes, "There is nothing to suggest that PED stories have any large overall negative impact with respect to how people view the game."[3]

> "There is nothing to suggest that PED stories have any large overall negative impact with respect to how people view the game."[3]
>
> —NBC Sports reporter Craig Calcaterra.

Reasons for Controversy

Regardless of how fans react, the issue of performance-enhancing drugs continues to cause controversy. Doctors warn about the harmful effects of anabolic steroids, which are synthetic male hormones that athletes use to build muscle mass and increase endurance. They say that short-term effects of steroid use include greater risk of high blood pressure, glaucoma, and fluid retention. Users also are prone to hormonal effects, such as mood swings, energy changes, and sleeplessness. Research indicates that the long-term use of steroids can lead to liver cancer, ruptured tendons, and lack of testosterone production. However, some fitness experts insist that steroids are basically safe if used in moderation. They point out that doctors prescribe steroids as treatment for certain inflammatory conditions, such as arthritis.

Another area of controversy is fairness in competition. Critics charge that PEDs give athletes an unfair advantage. They point to record-breaking performances that supposedly could only have been achieved with the help of drugs. Yet those who defend the use of PEDs counter that athletes have always sought to gain an edge over competitors. They claim there is often no great difference between acceptable diet supplements and banned PEDs. Some even recommend that rules about PED use be dropped entirely. There is also controversy over the regulation of PEDs at all levels of sport, from high school athletics to Olympic competition. As drug tests become more sophisticated, so too do athletes' and trainers' attempts to foil them.

It seems inevitable that the amazing breakthroughs of medical science and drug technology will find their way into sports competition, both amateur and professional. Even the weekend athlete or workout enthusiast can be tempted to try performance-enhancing drugs. As a result the debate over the harmful effects of PEDs will doubtless continue to rage.

What Are the Facts?

After months of denials, New York Yankees' slugger Alex Rodriguez (known popularly as A-Rod) confessed under oath in November 2014 that he indeed had used illegal steroids. Rodriguez, at the time baseball's highest-paid player, was testifying after a promise of immunity from federal prosecutors. He admitted to buying the performance-enhancing drugs from Anthony Bosch, a bogus doctor and owner of a Miami, Florida, firm called Biogenesis of America. It was Bosch who gave Rodriguez syringes prefilled with steroids for injections into his stomach. Rodriguez had always insisted defiantly that he had never taken PEDs—and not once had he failed a drug test. Yet his about-face before the grand jury revealed a pattern of using substances banned by MLB. Besides the syringes, Rodriguez had obtained other PED products, including lozenges and creams laced with testosterone. "Few sports fans have ever believed his innocence," says sports reporter Sean Gregory. "But his posturing looks so noxious now."[4] Cases like A-Rod's understandably reinforce a cynical attitude among sports fans. There is a tendency to assume that the most successful athletes are bound to be using PEDs. Yet many fans have only a vague idea about what performance-enhancing drugs are and how widespread their usage is among professional athletes and amateurs.

PEDs by the Numbers

Because most PEDs, such as anabolic steroids, are illegal without a doctor's prescription, statistics on their use can be sketchy and inconclusive. What is known is mostly based on anecdotal evidence and anonymous surveys. For example, a 2012 article in *Forbes* magazine claimed that PED use in professional sports is so widespread today that it is the new "normal." A 2009 poll of ex-NFL players suggested that about one in ten used steroids and that rates were even higher among offensive and defensive linemen. A German study of doping among elite athletes in all sports

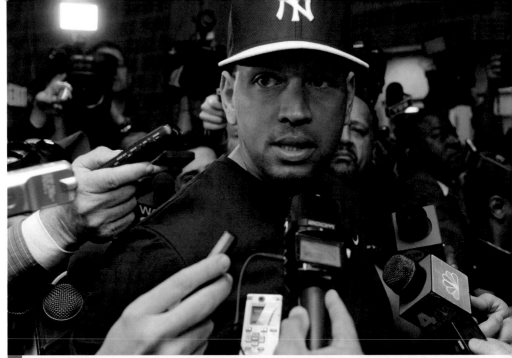

After issuing multiple denials, New York Yankees third baseman Alex Rodriguez (pictured here on Opening Day in 2013) abruptly reversed himself and admitted to having used illegal steroids. Admissions of PED use among top-tier athletes lead many sports fans to assume that any extraordinarily successful player must be using the substances.

found that 10.2 percent admitted to doping and another 24.7 percent cheated but lied about it. Most studies indicate that males are more than twice as likely to abuse steroids as females are. Adults from age eighteen to thirty-four are also twice as likely to have used steroids compared to the general population. As many as 1,084,000 Americans—about 0.5 percent of the adult population—admit to having used anabolic steroids, and the actual number of users is probably much higher.

Among high school students, research suggests that up to 12 percent of males and 1 percent of females have used anabolic steroids by the time they are seniors. Some 44 percent of young users say it is very easy or fairly easy for them to obtain steroids without a doctor's prescription. Four out of ten teenage users say they were influenced to take PEDs because professional athletes use them.

> "Few sports fans have ever believed [Alex Rodriguez's] innocence, but his posturing looks so noxious now."[4]
>
> —Sports reporter Sean Gregory.

PED Use Among Weekend Warriors

Professional athletes are not the only ones abusing PEDs. In April 2015, an international police group announced there is a greater public health concern about steroid use among so-called weekend warriors than among pro sports figures. Weekend warriors—a term often used mockingly—are amateur athletes and fitness enthusiasts who squeeze their exercise regimens into weekend games, runs, or workouts. Clément de Maillard, an antidoping officer at the International Criminal Police Organization (INTERPOL) believes these people have become the largest consumers of anabolic steroids and PEDs. "Actually this is a big health issue," says de Maillard. "We can consider the doping of professional athletes a kind of fraud, but regarding the mass consumption [of PEDs], it must be seen as a public health issue."

Experts attribute the growth in PED use among weekend warriors to the steroid culture in local gyms and easy availability of PEDs on the Internet. Whereas in years past, obtaining steroids required special contacts that only pro athletes or high-profile amateurs had, today anyone with a computer can order them via a Google search and a few clicks. Most of these drugs—excluding anabolic steroids, which require a doctor's prescription—are not illegal to possess or consume. Information about the use of PEDs and how to administer the drugs is also easy to find online. This extends to blood doping agents such as EPO that aid in endurance. Perhaps the middle-aged winner of the local 5K race owes his or her success to PEDs.

Quoted in Brian Blickenstaff, "The New Doping Crisis Is Not a Sports Issue, It's a Public Health Issue," *Vice Sports*, April 10, 2015. https://sports.vice.com.

Anti-PED Policies

Use of PEDs is banned at virtually every level of athletics, from professional leagues to college programs to high school teams. Every major sports league in America has its own policy on drug testing and specific penalties for PED use. For its part, MLB tests its players at least twice a year—once in spring training and once at a random date later in the season. Currently a player's first positive test for steroids results in an automatic suspension for 80 games without pay. A second positive test earns a full-season, 162-game suspension. A third positive test results in a lifetime ban. Since the MLB policy was implemented, thirty-nine players have been suspended, including stars like outfielder Ryan Braun and pitcher Ervin Santana. In the NFL, a first-time PED offense earns a suspension of up to six games (in a sixteen-game regular season). A second offense may result in a suspension of one year.

PEDs are also banned in college athletics, although enforcement is far from consistent. In general each school polices its own athletes and levies its own penalties for violations. The National Collegiate Athletics Association (NCAA) is seeking to bring greater oversight to the problem, but a program of standardized drug testing is still years away. PED use is illegal for high-school athletes as well, but drug testing is rare for high-school teams. Only about 20 percent of schools nationwide conduct tests for PEDs. "There are school districts that do conduct limited drug testing, but in terms of nationally, it's not very common,"[5] says Annie Skinner, spokeswoman for the US Anti-Doping Agency (USADA), which manages drug testing for the US Olympic teams. In fact, aside from the high-profile professional sports leagues, the blanket ban on PED use in American athletics is actually a patchwork of policies that allows many offenders to escape detection.

Statistics show that increasing numbers of high-school athletes are turning to PEDs as a shortcut to success on the field or court—this despite the fact that sale or possession of PEDs is illegal unless prescribed by a doctor. A 2014 survey by the Partnership for Drug-Free Kids showed high school athletes' use of synthetic human growth hormone having doubled from the previous year. Experts warn that too many teenagers view PED use as a normal aspect of strength training or bodybuilding.

> "There are school districts that do conduct limited drug testing [for PEDs], but in terms of nationally, it's not very common."[5]
>
> —Annie Skinner, spokeswoman for the US Anti-Doping Agency.

In Search of a Competitive Edge

Whether pros or aspiring amateurs, athletes use PEDs mainly to get a competitive edge. As early as the 1904 Olympics in

St. Louis, Missouri, American marathon runner Thomas Hicks used a dose of strychnine in brandy to revive in midrace and win the gold medal. Performance-enhancing drugs first gained wider attention in the 1930s with the discovery of how synthetic hormones, called steroids, could increase muscle mass and endurance and speed recovery from injuries. Over the next twenty years experiments with steroids increased among athletes, particularly those in the Soviet Union and Eastern Bloc countries. Impressed by these nations' dominant performance in weightlifting competition in the 1952 Olympics, US Olympic team physician Dr. John Ziegler began to issue steroids to American athletes. At Ziegler's urging, US chemists soon developed a steroid compound aimed at building strength with fewer side effects than the Soviet drug. The new steroid, called Dianabol, was the first to receive Food and Drug Administration (FDA) approval.

As steroid use expanded, sports officials moved to ban them as being potentially unsafe and providing an unfair advantage in competition. In the 1976 Montreal Olympics, the amazing success of the East German women's track and swim teams was found to be the result of doping. Trainers had given the so-called Wonder Girls vitamin pills that were actually steroids. At the 1988 Games in Seoul, South Korea, Canadian gold-medal-winning sprinter Ben Johnson's disqualification for steroid use brought unprecedented attention to the problem worldwide. In 1991 the US government passed laws that classed steroids as a controlled substance that could only be possessed legally under a doctor's prescription. Since the turn of the twenty-first century, regulators at international sports organizations and professional leagues have struggled to keep pace with the bewildering variety of compounds produced by steroid manufacturers and the many schemes to mask their use. The drive to get the slightest edge from drug use can prompt athletes to go to extraordinary lengths to foil mandatory drug tests.

The Science of Steroids

Although steroids are only one of the banned or illegal substances that sports-based drug tests are designed to detect, they are doubtless the most frequently used. When critics raise the issue of performance-enhancing drugs, they are generally referring to steroids or some form of hormonal supplement. Anabolic steroids are the synthetic version of the male sex hormone testosterone. Natural testosterone is produced by males almost exclusively in Leydig cells of the testes and by females in the ovaries. Production of testosterone in males is about ten times the level

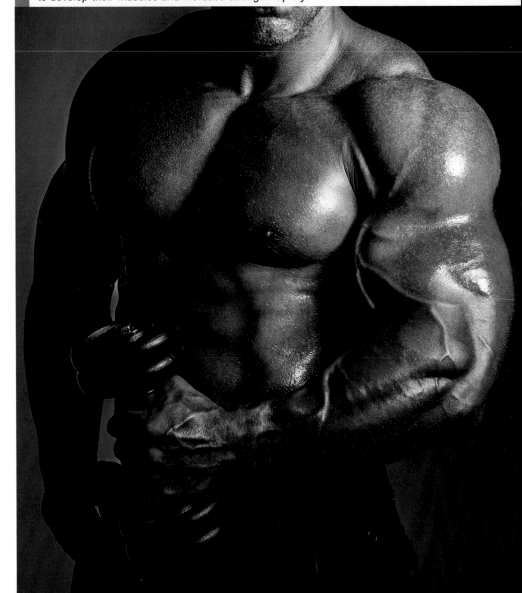

A bodybuilder shows off his muscles. Although anabolic-androgenic steroids have many legitimate medical uses, athletes and bodybuilders of both sexes take them to develop their muscles and increase strength rapidly.

in females. With age, a male's level of testosterone production declines continuously. Anabolic steroids take the place of naturally produced testosterone, dampening the body's production of and disrupting the internal balance of that hormone.

The full technical name for human-made steroids is anabolic-androgenic steroids. *Anabolic* means they promote bone strength and muscle growth. This results from stimulating receptor molecules in bone and muscle cells, which in turn activate specific genes to produce proteins. The synthesis of muscle protein helps athletes increase their strength. *Androgenic* means the steroids enhance the development of male sexual characteristics—such as excess growth of body hair, oily skin and acne, and deepening voice—in both male and female users. Doctors prescribe anabolic steroids to treat various conditions, including hormone deficiency, anemia, burns, cancer, and AIDS. For athletes and bodybuilders, anabolic steroids have no medical purpose but are used to improve performance or physical appearance.

Athletes take anabolic steroids to develop their muscles and increase strength more quickly. This occurs because steroids reduce the body's levels of cortisol, a powerful hormone that is released by the adrenal glands under conditions of stress. Cortisol increases blood sugar and regulates the immune system. It tends to have a catabolic effect, breaking down muscle tissue, controlling inflammation, and storing fat to protect the body. Reducing cortisol helps athletes build muscle mass and increase their strength dramatically. "Essentially, anabolic steroids induce a second adolescence," says Dr. Charles Yesalis, professor of health policy and sport science at Penn State University. "Many of the same things happen as would in puberty. As testosterone levels elevate, the user experiences increased strength and muscle mass. In a sport like baseball, that strength makes it easier to hit a home run, with stronger forearms to power through the ball and powerful hips to rotate your body quickly."[6] Steroids allow for more intense training regimens and more rapid recovery afterward. In endurance sports, this can provide a decisive edge. Anabolic steroids are also used to hasten recovery from injury.

Most forms of anabolic steroids, including Dianabol, Stanozolol, Trenbolone, and Winstrol, are taken orally or injected into muscles. Some, such as tetrahydrogestrinone, or THG, work by being applied to the skin as a cream or gel. In general, the doses that athletes and bodybuilders take are ten to one hundred times greater than those prescribed for medical treatment. These users generally take steroids intermittently instead of continuously, in a use pattern called cycling. Continuous use can lessen the body's response to the drugs and also can shut down the body's own production of testosterone. Cycling restricts use of anabolic steroids to a few weeks or months at a time, after which the user completely stops taking the drugs for a certain period before resuming use. With the advent of many different types of steroids and hormone supplements, users often combine several in their training regime, a practice known as stacking.

Mental and Physical Effects of Steroid Abuse

Many athletes, bodybuilders, and weekend users consider steroids to be merely training supplements rather than dangerous substances. Nonetheless steroid abusers can experience changes in brain pathways and chemicals much like those associated with addiction. Users may spend lots of money and time in obtaining steroids—a telltale addictive behavior—and may continue using them despite their adverse effects on the users' health and social life. Steroid abuse can also cause psychiatric problems and mood swings. Not uncommon are steroid-related episodes of extreme aggression and anger—a condition known as "roid rage." Other psychological effects include irritability, irrational jealousy, delusions, and impaired judgment related to feelings of being invincible. Once users stop taking steroids, they can suffer withdrawal symptoms, including depression and suicidal thoughts, fatigue, insomnia, loss of appetite, and cravings for the drugs.

"Essentially, anabolic steroids induce a second adolescence. Many of the same things happen as would in puberty."[6]

—Dr. Charles Yesalis, professor of health policy and sport science at Penn State University.

Athletes and bodybuilders who use anabolic steroids tend to take them at very high doses. It would be unethical to conduct tests on athletes by intentionally giving them such high doses of steroids. Thus information about the physical effects of anabolic steroids is mostly limited to case reports on users. Nonetheless certain adverse physical effects are well documented. Since steroid abuse disrupts the normal production of testosterone, it can cause temporary effects on parts of the body that rely on the regulation of this hormone. These effects may include reduced sperm production, impotence, and shrinking of the testicles, as well as long-term changes such as male-pattern baldness and breast development in men. Women may develop a deeper voice and experience infrequent or absent menstrual periods. Children or adolescents using anabolic steroids can prematurely limit bone growth, while adults can suffer ruptured tendons. Cardiovascular effects from steroid abuse include high blood pressure, fluid retention, enlargement of the heart, and increased risk of heart attack, blood clots, and atherosclerosis (hardened arteries). Steroid abuse is also linked to liver tumors and a rare condition in which blood-filled cysts form in the liver. In addition, taking steroids via a shared needle greatly increases risk of bacterial infections or serious viral infections such as HIV and hepatitis B and C.

Other Types of PEDs

Although anabolic steroids are the most frequently abused PED, there are many other types. Some are similar to steroids in their effects and others are targeted to improve specific areas of performance. Human growth hormone (HGH) is used to build muscle mass and recover from injuries in a way similar to steroids. Produced in the pituitary gland, HGH stimulates the release of proteins from the liver that trigger the building of cartilage in body tissues. This results in the increase of bone and muscle cells in developing adolescents. HGH also helps regulate body fluids as well as sugar and fat metabolism. These developments remain largely active through young adulthood, but after the twenties, the amount of HGH begins to decline. Because adding HGH to the body can artificially compensate for the decline of the body's production, some promoters tout HGH supplements as anti-aging

Uppers for Energy

In 2014 two of Baltimore's star professional athletes, the Orioles' Chris Davis and the Ravens' Haloti Ngata, were suspended by their respective leagues (baseball and football) for use of the amphetamine Adderall. Sportswriters noted wryly that these bruising players had been caught sneaking a drug best known for its use in treating children for attention-deficit/hyperactivity disorder (ADHD). As *Baltimore Sun* reporter Childs Walker noted about Ngata, "The giant was felled for using a drug most often associated with being prescribed to children who can't sit still. Ngata will sit out the next four games—all vital to the Ravens' wavering playoff chances—for using Adderall." Neither Ngata nor Davis had an explanation for their actions, but presumably both were seeking a boost to their energy and alertness by using an amphetamine.

Also known as uppers or speed, amphetamines are nonsteroidal PEDs that stimulate the central nervous system and increase the user's energy level. Amphetamines include such drugs as Adderall, Benzedrine, and Dexedrine. Besides ADHD, they are sometimes prescribed for chronic fatigue or to treat a sleep disorder called narcolepsy. These drugs are similar in chemical structure to adrenaline, a stress hormone that is produced naturally in the body's adrenal glands. Athletes who take uppers seek improved reaction time and cognitive function as well as an increase in energy and alertness. Experts say the drugs' minor short-term benefits are generally outweighed by risks of addiction, cerebral hemorrhage, high blood pressure, angina, irritability and restlessness, and insomnia.

Childs Walker, "Ravens' Haloti Ngata Is the Latest Star Athlete Suspended for Using Adderall," *Baltimore Sun*, December 4, 2014. http://touch.baltimoresun.com.

products, but medical experts insist this claim is unproven. Synthetic HGH, developed in 1985, won FDA approval as a treatment for several medical conditions that limit body growth, such as the chromosomal disorder called Turner syndrome and the genetic illness called SHOX deficiency. HGH use has long been considered less dangerous than steroid use. The NFL began testing players for HGH only in 2014, and the National Basketball Association (NBA) in 2016. MLB has banned HGH since 2005, but some players question the policy. "If HGH were legal," says pitcher Ryan Madson, "just in the process of healing, under a doctor's recommendation, in the right dosage, while you're on the [disabled list], I don't think that's such a bad idea—as long as it doesn't have any lasting side effects, *negative* side effects."[7]

Androstenedione is another hormone-related substance that athletes use to develop muscle and speed recovery from injuries. Andro, as it is called, is a naturally occurring hormone produced by the adrenal glands that helps boost testosterone levels. Andro became famous in 1998 when reporters spotted a bottle of it in the locker of St. Louis Cardinals' slugger Mark McGwire, a discovery that led eventually to baseball's steroid scandal. In 2004 the FDA banned its sale, citing serious safety concerns.

"If HGH were legal, just in the process of healing, under a doctor's recommendation, in the right dosage, while you're on the [disabled list], I don't think that's such a bad idea."[7]

—MLB pitcher Ryan Madson.

Creatine is an organic acid that helps supply energy to the body's cells, particularly muscle cells. It has become one of the most popular over-the-counter supplements for weight gain and muscle development among athletes and bodybuilders. Taken usually as a flavored powder mixed with water, creatine can provide short-term bursts of energy for certain kinds of training, such as sprints and power lifting. The supplement has undergone many studies on its safety. "Creatine is one of the most-researched sports supplements out there," says Chad Kerksick, assistant professor of exercise physiology at the University of Oklahoma. "And there's no published literature to suggest it's unsafe."[8] Nonetheless there are persistent anecdotal reports of bad side effects, including kidney damage, heart problems, muscle cramps, dehydration, and diarrhea.

Endurance athletes such as cyclists and distance runners use an illegal technique called blood doping to improve performance. Blood doping boosts the number of red blood cells in the bloodstream to increase the flow of oxygen from the lungs to the muscles. A higher concentration of oxygen in the blood raises an athlete's aerobic capacity, enabling him or her to work

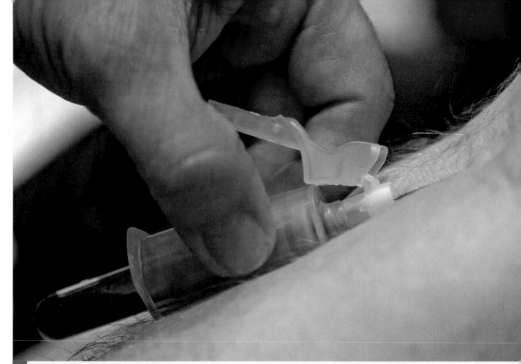

A doctor takes a blood sample as part of a demonstration of how antidoping agencies carry out their work. Blood tests may reveal that an athlete has been engaging in the practice of blood doping, or using illicit means to boost the number of red blood cells in the bloodstream. This increases the oxygen flow from the lungs to the muscles, enabling the athlete to work harder for a longer period than would otherwise be the case.

harder for a longer period. Blood doping is accomplished in three different ways. An athlete may have a unit of blood drawn, store it for three weeks while his body replaces the lost blood, and then have the unit transfused back into the bloodstream shortly before competition in order to get an infusion of red blood cells. The athlete may also receive a transfusion of someone else's blood of the same type. A second method involves injecting erythropoietin (EPO), a protein hormone produced by the kidney. Released into the bloodstream, EPO binds with receptors in the bone marrow to stimulate the production of red blood cells. Athletes inclined to cheat favor EPO as an improvement over messy transfusions and also because it is difficult to detect in testing. A third type of blood doping is the use of synthetic oxygen carriers. These are employed in emergency therapies when a patient needs a blood transfusion but there is no blood available, there is a high risk of blood infection, or there is no time for matching blood type. Like other forms of blood doping, synthetic oxygen carriers provide an athlete with a sudden oxygen boost in the bloodstream to keep muscles working longer at peak efficiency.

An Ongoing Problem

PEDS continue to lure athletes seeking peak performance in today's sports world. With skyrocketing salaries and TV contracts, the pressure to reach the top or remain competitive is intense. This pressure leads many athletes to abuse anabolic steroids or other PEDs. Scientists agree that more studies are needed to establish the facts about these substances and about other new drugs designed to enhance performance. The controversy over PEDs shows no signs of going away.

How Dangerous Is the Use of Performance-Enhancing Drugs?

Mike Matarazzo was one of the few professional bodybuilders of his time to speak openly about the sport's risks from the use of steroids and other drugs. "Most guys think nothing bad will ever happen to them," Matarazzo said about his fellow competitors. "But you watch. You'll be seeing more and more serious heart problems, and worse, once these guys hit 40."[9] Matarazzo's words became a self-fulfilling prophecy when he died in 2014 of complications related to steroid use. Originally trained as a boxer, he had years of success as a pro bodybuilder in the 1990s, with his massively muscled physique, crisscrossed with bulging veins, featured on dozens of magazine covers and websites.

> "Most guys think nothing bad will ever happen to them [from using PEDs]. But you watch. You'll be seeing more and more serious heart problems, and worse, once these guys hit 40."[9]
>
> —Mike Matarazzo, professional bodybuilder.

Soon however Matarazzo began to have serious cardiovascular problems that forced him to retire. In 2004 he experienced severely clogged arteries, a common reaction to excessive use of steroids and their increased production of red blood cells. Three years later, life-threatening complications caused him to undergo triple-bypass heart surgery. He was hoping for a heart transplant when he died at a Stanford University hospital. Yet in spite of Matarazzo's own testimony about steroid abuse, many followers of his sport refused to blame his death on PEDs. "To our amazement, bloggers on forums were in complete denial, attributing Mike's heart issues to secondary contributing factors such as high-fat diets, excessive protein intake, and other anomalies,"[10] writes MuscleK on the website Steroid Analysis.

The Dangers of Ignoring the Risks

For every pro bodybuilder with steroid-related heart disease, there are many more amateurs dealing with similar problems. Oli Cooney, an amateur from West Yorkshire, England, began his own fanatical bodybuilding program at age sixteen. Cooney took massive amounts of anabolic steroids in a quest to change his body image. By age eighteen, he was receiving warnings from doctors to limit his excessive exercise regime. Hospitalized with chest pains, Cooney was diagnosed with serious heart damage. Eventually he had two heart attacks and three strokes, leaving him unable to speak for a time and convincing him to stop using PEDs. Yet by that point the damage to Cooney's heart was irreversible. He ignored doctors' orders and returned to gym workouts several times a week. In 2014 Cooney collapsed and died after running to catch a taxi. He was only twenty years old. Dominic Bell, the local coroner, ruled Cooney's death the direct result of steroid abuse. "He had this weakness that he was driven to alter his body image to become more confident in society,"[11] said Bell.

> "The irony is that steroid users are often health-oriented, but they're using a drug that is damaging their bodies to the point it could kill. These men are doing major damage to their hearts and are substantially increasing their risk of death."[12]
>
> —Shane Darke, professor at the Australian national drug and alcohol research center at the University of New South Wales.

The deaths of bodybuilders like Matarazzo and Cooney underscore the findings of a recent study in Australia on steroid abuse. Researchers discovered that men in their late twenties and early thirties who abuse steroids run the risk of severe health problems, including cardiovascular disease, reproductive trouble, liver damage, and outbreaks of aggression. Researchers looked at twenty-four men who had died over a period of seventeen years in steroid-related episodes. The men worked as personal trainers, security guards, and bodybuilders. Nearly all of them showed major signs of steroid abuse, such as overdeveloped muscles, shrunken and scarred testicles, and the thickened arteries and damaged heart muscle associated with cardiovascular disease. Despite the men's focus on fitness—often to the point of obsession—they were willing to use drugs that did obvious damage to their bodies. According to study leader Shane Darke, a professor at the Australian national drug and alcohol research center at the University of New South Wales:

The irony is that steroid users are often health-oriented, but they're using a drug that is damaging their bodies to the point it could kill. These men are doing major damage to their hearts and are substantially increasing their risk of death. For a very young group in their early 30s, their cardiac health looks like what you would expect of someone twice their age.[12]

Darke notes that while most steroid users are probably aware of certain side effects, most seem oblivious to the risks of heart disease. Generally fitness enthusiasts do not consider PEDs to be drugs in the same sense as heroin or cocaine. It is important, he says, to get the message out that taking steroids is not a healthy option, that in fact these are dangerous drugs capable of causing serious damage.

This photo shows an artery clogged by a deposit of cholesterol known as plaque. Severely clogged arteries are only one of the cardiovascular problems that can result from steroid use.

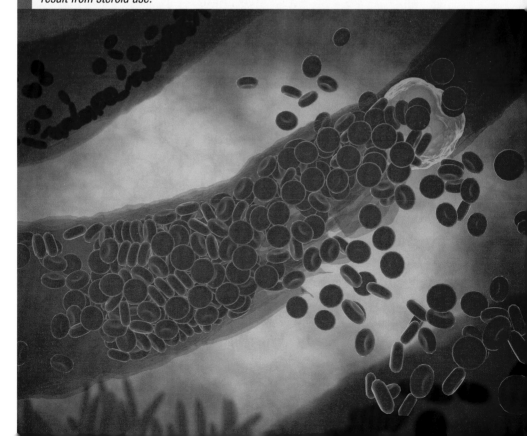

Long-Term Physical Effects

Many bodybuilders and athletes who use anabolic steroids think they can avoid negative side effects through cycling—alternating periods of use and nonuse—combined with supplements to restore hormonal balance. What they fail to realize is how serious are the long-term effects of the drugs, both physiological and psychological. Physiological side effects refer to changes in the body's functions and activities. Specifically this concerns the organs, tissues, and cells and all the chemical reactions between and among them. Appearance-related effects of steroid use such as acne and excess body hair pale in comparison to the permanent physiological effects. These, if left untreated, can cause serious health problems and even threaten the user's life.

Certain systems of the body are directly impacted by abuse of anabolic steroids. For example, the ability of steroids to strengthen

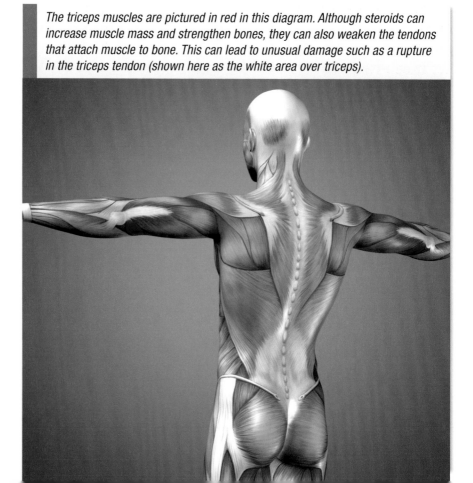

The triceps muscles are pictured in red in this diagram. Although steroids can increase muscle mass and strengthen bones, they can also weaken the tendons that attach muscle to bone. This can lead to unusual damage such as a rupture in the triceps tendon (shown here as the white area over triceps).

bones and increase muscle mass is well known, but they also cause a weakening of tendons that attach muscle to bone. The elastic fibers of tendons are mainly made of collagen. Anabolic steroids disrupt the formation of normal collagen fibrils, which make up the fibers in tendons, within a few days after being introduced to a person's system. Instead, the drugs cause the production of abnormal fibrils that greatly increase in size with exercise. The result is stiffer tendons with much less tensile strength. An extreme motion, such as a power lift or sudden shift of direction while sprinting, can easily rupture such a tendon. When an athletic trainer sees severe or unusual tendon damage, such as a rupture of the triceps tendon in the upper arm, he or she immediately suspects steroid use. Repeated damage to minor tendons is also common with steroid users. The resulting accumulated scar tissue and weakened tendon links can sideline an athlete for months and eventually end his or her career.

Anabolic steroids often increase bone production, particularly in the skull and face. As the maxilla and mandible (upper and lower jaws, respectively) expand, teeth can splay apart. Some users experience an overgrown forehead, which can look much like that of the comics character the Hulk. With adolescent teenagers who are still growing, steroid abuse can prematurely close bone-growth plates and limit their stature. This occurs when the steroid stimulates bone growth to outstrip cartilage production between the plates and seals the plates more rigidly together.

Steroid abuse can also throw the male reproductive system out of balance, suppressing the body's natural production of testosterone. Studies differ on whether hormonal balance and testicular function can be restored to normal after steroid use is discontinued. Some research suggests hormonal problems may persist even after stoppage of the drugs.

Whereas direct links between anabolic steroids and fatal heart disease have been hard to establish, most experts agree that steroid abuse contributes to cardiovascular disease, including heart attacks and strokes. This happens partly because steroids change the levels of lipoproteins, the molecules that carry cholesterol in the blood. Anabolic steroids, particularly those taken

Steroids Are Dangerous for Both Adults and Adolescents

The health risks associated with using anabolic steroids are well established, says baseball historian and writer William C. Kashatus. He argues that both adults and young people need to be aware of the dangers.

PEDs taken in megadoses have been linked to tendon and ligament tears, kidney and liver damage, impotence, heart disease and cancer.

Unlike pro athletes, teenagers are more susceptible to the physiological and psychological effects of steroids because of the natural hormonal imbalance. The effects include irritability, rage, depression and suicidal tendencies. . . .

There is a desperate need for greater awareness of the dangers and symptoms of steroid use among adults. Unfortunately, most parents cannot distinguish between those symptoms and the extreme mood swings, severe acne and physical maturation associated with adolescence. . . .

Regardless of one's position, there is no denying the fact that steroids are illegal. Their sale and use without a physician's prescription is a felony. Scientists, doctors and lawmakers long ago decided that steroids are so dangerous that they must be subject to medical and legal control. . . .

It's time for parents, coaches and the professional athletes who, whether they like it or not, are role models for our kids, to take greater responsibility on this issue. If we fail, we have nobody to blame but ourselves.

William C. Kashatus, "Dangers of Steroid Use Are Real," Chron, June 17, 2013. www.chron.com.

orally, tend to increase the user's level of low-density lipoprotein (LDL), also known as bad cholesterol. They stimulate a liver enzyme that reduces high-density lipoprotein (HDL), or the so-called good cholesterol that helps remove LDL and eliminate plaque deposits in the arteries. Reduced HDL increases risk of atherosclerosis, or arteries blocked by fatty substances that disrupt healthy blood flow. Such blockages can lead to heart attack or stroke.

Anabolic steroids also cause users to retain fluids, which contributes to high blood pressure. Over time, steroid use combined with rigorous training can lead to an enlarged heart and a decrease

The Dangers of Anabolic Steroids Are Exaggerated

There are medical experts, like Dr. Charles E. Yesalis, who insist that the risks of steroid use have been exaggerated. Yesalis, a professor at Penn State University and consultant to the NFL Players Association, says steroids are mainly harmful if misused.

> There are some drugs on the list [of banned substances in MLB] where we don't have really hardcore evidence that they enhance performance. . . . Our data on growth hormone, even though I personally believe that it is a performance enhancer, you look at some of the studies they've done, and it's unclear. Then another factor is safety. Some drugs like anabolic steroids and growth hormone, especially steroids, I don't know if they're all that dangerous. They're clearly not a major killer drug like amphetamines can be, or cocaine, or heroin, or tobacco for that matter. So for a long time those of us who are observers of this scene, the rationale for putting a drug on [the list of banned substances] is often not that clear and consistent. . . .
>
> If you take anabolic steroids in high doses for protracted periods of time it's difficult to think you could fool mother nature, that some adverse effects will not befall you. But they're not what I'd call major killer drugs. We use them in medicine, and I'd hope we're not purposefully killing our patients.

Quoted in Pack Bringley, "Explaining Steroids: Interview with a PED Expert," *Amazin' Avenue* (blog), SB Nation, August 6, 2013. www.amazinavenue.com.

VIEWPOINT

in the heart's pumping ability. Anabolic steroids can harm liver function as well. Abuse of the drugs is associated with liver tumors, both benign and malignant, and blood-filled cysts on the liver, which can rupture and cause dangerous internal bleeding.

Emotional and Behavioral Effects

With all the emphasis on how anabolic steroids can ravage the body, their effect on a user's mind is often overlooked. Although the science of these effects is still unclear, the mental changes can be as harmful in their way as the physical damage. Users frequently report episodes of manic rage while on the drugs—incidents sometimes called "roid rage." Feelings of extreme aggressiveness may be useful for competitive athletes such as linebackers or mixed martial arts fighters, but they can also result in violent and even criminal behavior. For example, in June 2007, Canadian pro wrestler Chris Benoit murdered his wife and son before hanging himself. Reports of Benoit's longtime steroid use led to speculation that the drugs contributed to his actions.

Under the influence of steroids, users can become disconnected from reality. They may feel invincible, with an urgent need to prove themselves if challenged. They may not even be aware of how their behavior is changing. Some researchers believe the drugs mainly intensify the aggression that comes naturally to the competitive types who take them. According to Dr. Gary Wadler, member of WADA and author of *Drugs and the Athlete*,

> "Roid rage, in many ways, I would characterize as a form of loss of impulse control. . . . Forget the roid, for the moment. It's a rage . . . and that rage is precipitated by the brain being exposed to anabolic steroids."[13]
>
> —Dr. Gary Wadler, member of the World Anti-Doping Agency and author of *Drugs and the Athlete*.

Roid rage, in many ways, I would characterize as a form of loss of impulse control. So say somebody says something to you that you don't like. You may put your fist through a wall. The impulse is there; it's overreaction. Forget the roid, for the moment. It's a rage . . . and that rage is precipitated by the brain being exposed to anabolic steroids.[13]

Another common emotional effect of using anabolic steroids is depression. In some cases users may become suicidal. Those taking the drugs because of issues they have with their own body image may be particularly prone to depression. Users might also take other drugs to ease their steroid-related depression or cure their sleeplessness, which can worsen the cycle of abuse.

Hazards of Other PEDs

Anabolic steroids are not the only PEDs that pose health dangers. Overuse of the hormone HGH can increase risks of cancer and diabetes and also cause joint pain, vision problems, fluid retention, high blood pressure, and an enlarged heart. HGH was once considered a promising anti-aging treatment,

This X-ray shows an enlarged heart pictured in red. An enlarged heart can result from overuse of human growth hormone (HGH), a PED that athletes use to build muscle mass and reduce recovery time from injuries.

and many older individuals still take it to improve skin appearance and muscle tone. But some studies show that higher levels of growth hormone in older adults can actually reduce longevity. "Overwhelmingly the human data and the research and the science will say that, for the majority of people, [taking HGH is] just a bad idea,"[14] says Valter Longo, director of the Longevity Institute at the University of Southern California.

Using EPO to stimulate production of red blood cells is also hazardous. EPO use among competitive cyclists in the 1990s is blamed for at least eighteen deaths. Injections of EPO thicken the blood and increase the strain on a user's heart, particularly during downtime or sleep when the heart rate slows. Increased blood thickness raises the risk of blood clots, heart attacks, and strokes. According to cycling expert Matt Rendell, some cyclists in the Tour de France bike race would set an alarm each night to wake up and peddle on a training bike for ten minutes to jump-start their circulatory system and lessen the risks from their use of EPO.

Amphetamines are another class of drugs whose short-term benefits for athletes are outweighed by health risks. Even moderate use of amphetamines can distort the user's perception of pain or fatigue, leading him or her to ignore warning signs of serious injury. Long-term abuse can lead to dependency, high blood pressure and heart rate, sleeplessness, weight loss, feelings of anxiety and irritability, and greater risk of heart attack and kidney failure. A. Marc Gillinov, a heart surgeon and author of a book on heart health, is candid about the dangers of PEDs: "When it comes to PEDs, let's recognize their health risks and add an additional word, making the goal 'Fair, Safe Play.'"[15]

Weighing Risks Against Positive Factors

Despite all the evidence about the dangers of PEDs, there are some who insist the risks are overblown and should be weighed against positive factors. Medical experts acknowledge that anabolic steroids and HGH have many legitimate uses. Dr. John Baxter, a professor in the metabolic research unit at UC San Francisco, believes the idea that hormone supplements "are equivalent to taking heroin or something is unfair. . . . The thing that disturbs me is that we seem to be demonizing something that for many people could have great therapeutic benefit."[16]

Baxter was referring mainly to older men with lower levels of testosterone, but doctors refer to other positive effects every day. Supporters point out that the FDA has approved many growth hormone products for patients who have chronically low levels of testosterone. In addition, proper use of steroids in regulated doses can assist in healing muscle injuries and restoring strength. Anabolic steroids are often prescribed for short-term use to help patients gain weight after a severe illness or injury or when they are suffering from an unexplained weight loss. Some patients may also be in need of increased muscle mass and bone density, and steroids can help accomplish this. They also are used to treat certain kinds of anemia. Corticosteroids, a more common group, are useful in reducing inflammation and controlling the immune system. For this reason, they can treat asthma, arthritis, autoimmune diseases, skin conditions, and certain types of cancer.

> "Think about it: medical science has been using steroids safely in a clinical setting for the last 70 years."[17]
>
> —Dr. Charles Yesalis, consultant to the NFL Players Association and the US Olympic Committee.

Steroid use today is not limited to elite athletes and bodybuilders. The Mayo Clinic estimates that 3 million people in the United States take anabolic steroids. Easy availability via gyms and mail order has made usage among young people very popular. Some experts believe these statistics argue in favor of the drugs' relative safety, especially if used in low doses and monitored closely. They point out that up until 2004 over-the-counter dietary supplements such as Andro and THG could be obtained without prescription in health food stores. "Think about it: medical science has been using steroids safely in a clinical setting for the last 70 years," says Dr. Charles Yesalis, a leading expert on PEDs and a consultant to the NFL Players Association and the US Olympic Committee. "Anabolic steroids can be used relatively safely, but at even low doses they can have side effects. No drug, supplement, or substance is totally 'safe.'"[17]

There are also physicians who question the hazards of blood-doping drugs like EPO. Peter Janssen, former team doctor with the Vacansoleil pro cycling team, argues that the banned drug is actually harmless and says he would recommend its use for the safety of riders in a long, grueling race. "If my son was a professional cyclist and had to ride a Grand Tour like the Giro d'Italia right now, I would accompany him on the trip and make sure that he sometimes got a little EPO," says Janssen. "Not to increase his chance of winning, but simply to maintain his health."[18]

The Consensus About PEDs

The opinions of Janssen and Yesalis place them in a tiny minority compared to the consensus views about PEDs among doctors and medical professionals. Janssen, for example, even denies the increased risk of blood clots, stroke, and heart attack from EPO use, despite reams of evidence to the contrary. The fact that there are almost no detailed clinical studies on PED abuse—mainly because of the risks to the subjects' long-term health—can lead some to downplay the dangers of these drugs. Nonetheless, most doctors agree the hazards of using PEDs are real and can easily become life threatening.

Should Performance-Enhancing Drugs Be Illegal?

On December 18, 2015, a sweeping new antidoping law took effect in Germany. The law provides that athletes who test positive for performance-enhancing drugs or are found in possession of such drugs can face prison terms of up to three years. Individuals who help athletes procure PEDs, including doctors, coaches, or fellow athletes, would face prison sentences of up to ten years. The law targets professional athletes, not amateurs, and includes offenders visiting from other nations as well as German citizens.

While possession of PEDs was already a crime in Germany, the new law focuses on usage. It is part of a growing hard-line approach to the problem in Germany, coming a few months after the German Football (Soccer) Association announced plans to give its players blood tests for doping on match days. According to interior minister Thomas de Maiziere, the new legislation is long overdue. "I am convinced that we can tackle doping in sport and the criminal structures behind it more effectively with this anti-doping law," says de Maiziere, who also described it as "a clear commitment of Germany for clean and fair sport."[19] Some critics also wanted a provision so courts could grant leniency to key witnesses in hopes they would testify against offenders who conspire together in groups. It was hoped that this would help uncover so-called doping networks like the one that supported American cyclist Lance Armstrong. Nonetheless, the new German antidoping law promises to be a model of tighter regulation for other countries in Europe and around the world.

Laws Regulating PEDs

The new German antidoping law is also significant because it represents the policy of the government, not just separate sports organizations. Many believe the key to solving the problem of PEDs in sports is for national governments to adopt tougher laws. In the 2013 World Conference on Doping in Sport, Olympic Committee president Dr. Thomas Bach urged nations to pass strict laws and increase their cooperation in doping cases. "We need a better exchange of information between state authorities, the sports movement and the national anti-doping organizations," Bach said. "This also means that the state authorities must do more to severely punish those behind the scenes in doping cases: the dealers, the agents, coaches, doctors, scientists and all other involved in doping activities."[20] For Bach, catching and penalizing athletes who dope is important above all for the protection of clean athletes, who are tainted by the association with drug use. When athletes succeed with the help of PEDs, fans mistakenly assume that all the competitors must be doping to some extent, unfairly lumping clean athletes in with those who are taking the drugs.

Some see Germany's crackdown on PED use as a sign the antidoping movement is gaining force. Yet the legal status of PEDs varies widely from country to country. Australia, Argentina, Brazil,

The German Football (Soccer) Association requires its players (dressed in white) to submit to blood tests for doping on match days. A few months after the association established this rule, German legislators passed a law that made testing positive for PEDs a crime punishable by up to three years in prison.

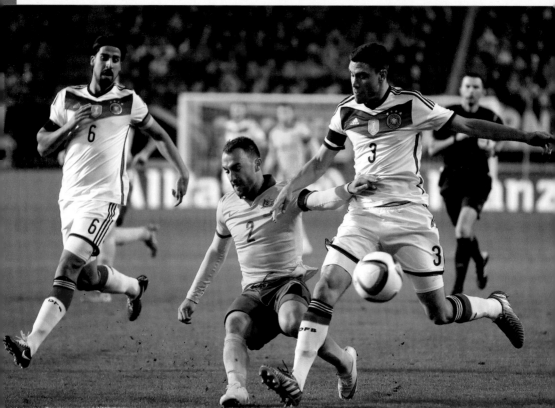

Canada, and Portugal require a doctor's prescription for legal purchase of anabolic steroids. A majority of nations, however, either have no laws against PEDs or ones that are very lax. For example, in Great Britain and most European countries anabolic steroids can be purchased in a pharmacy much like a bottle of cough syrup. Many nations, including Colombia, Egypt, India, Russia, Mexico, and Thailand, place no limits on buying, selling, possessing, or manufacturing steroids. Mexico's lenient policy attracts many American buyers, although the drugs cannot legally be brought back across the border.

In the United States many PEDs are classified as a controlled substance. Anabolic steroids have been regulated under the Controlled Substances Act since 1990. Possession of anabolic steroids without a valid prescription is a federal crime that carries a maximum penalty of one year in prison and a fine of $1,000. The maximum penalty for trafficking the drugs is five years in prison and a fine of $250,000. Second offenses result in double the imprisonment time and fine amounts. Similar penalties apply to HGH and other types of designer steroids. These substances are illegal without a prescription under both federal and state law in the United States. Most PED-related crimes are actually prosecuted at the state level, where fines and jail terms vary widely.

A number of PEDs, such as the blood-doping drug EPO, are legal by prescription in the United States but are banned by sports organizations. The WADA, established in 1999 by the International Olympic Committee, is the main nongovernmental body fighting drugs in sports. It maintains a list of banned substances that is ten pages long and includes everything from prescription drugs to stimulants and painkillers found in over-the-counter medicines. Although American pro sports leagues are not governed by the WADA, they do consult with the group in designing their testing programs for illegal substances. In December 2015, controversial allegations about PED use by high-profile stars of pro football and pro baseball in the United States brought public statements of concern by WADA officials. "In recent years WADA has been working with [the NFL and MLB] and other professional leagues in the United States to try to bring them closer to WADA's program," said David Howman, director general of the WADA. "We would of course welcome increased collaboration with the leagues and their players' associations to discuss appropriate enhancements that could be made in support of clean athletes."[21]

Policy as a Deterrent

The main reason that many PEDs are illegal in the United States and banned by groups like the WADA is the health danger they present. Relatively little research has been done about the long-term effects of anabolic steroids and other PEDs, but there is plenty of anecdotal evidence about their risks and dangers. Experts admit that elite athletes may not be deterred by these risks.

In their drive to succeed, athletes are willing to try almost anything, both in training and competition. Pro players, faced with limited career spans, may balance the health risks of using PEDs with their need to maintain an edge and protect their livelihood. From this perspective the most that today's antidoping laws and policies can do is help curb the use of PEDs, not prevent it. Should PEDs be legalized, however, some fear there would be a sort of "arms race" to develop more and more potent substances. All the resources of modern chemistry and biology would be deployed, as indeed they have been recently in sports such as cycling. Athletes would become guinea pigs, willingly or not, in their use of untested and potentially deadly new drugs. Therefore, critics maintain that antidoping laws are necessary roadblocks to keep PED development and use from spiraling out of control.

> "There appears to be a widespread misconception that PED use is primarily a phenomenon among a small group of highly competitive elite athletes. . . . PED use is not limited to elite athletes but involves a much larger group of nonathlete weightlifters."[22]
>
> —Harrison G. Pope and a research group for the Endocrine Society.

Fears About Unregulated Sales

Laws against certain PEDs also help protect the amateur athlete and so-called weekend warrior. As a research group for the Endocrine Society reports, "There appears to be a widespread misconception

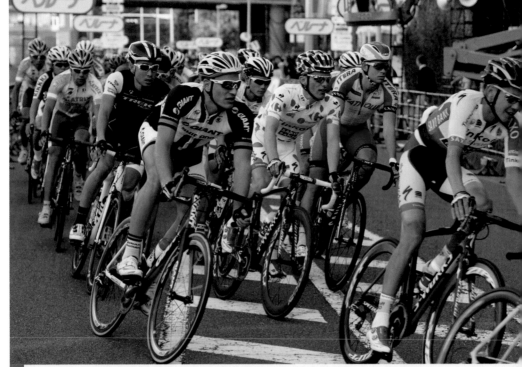

Cyclists race in the Tour de France Saitama Critérium competition in Japan. The sport of cycling has weathered several doping scandals, leading many observers to view unexpected or atypical athletic performances with suspicion that they were achieved with PED use.

that PED use is primarily a phenomenon among a small group of highly competitive elite athletes. This misperception has distracted attention from the health risks associated with PED use and the fact that PED use is not limited to elite athletes but involves a much larger group of nonathlete weightlifters."[22] As the group notes, the vast majority of PED users are not professional athletes or even competitive athletes at all. Instead they are weightlifters and bodybuilders who follow their own workout program and take the drugs without a doctor's supervision. These individuals often become obsessive in their use of anabolic steroids and HGH, taking them in dangerously high doses and neglecting to cycle off the drugs to give their bodies a rest. A significant percentage of young PED users also take other drugs, including opioids, cocaine, or ecstasy. Among nonathlete users, testing for PEDs is almost nonexistent, making regulation of their usage that much more difficult. With PEDs obtainable online, in gyms, and from mail-order sellers, no law, however well intended, is able to prevent weekend warriors from using PEDs. Nevertheless,

Legalizing PEDs Would Lead to Safer Usage

PEDs should be legal as long as they are used at medically acceptable levels, says Kate Schmidt, former US Olympic javelin thrower. She believes that legalizing PEDs would actually help prevent their abuse.

What if we decriminalized and destigmatized performance-enhancing drugs—indeed, called them "training supplements"? . . . By accepting these currently banned substances as mainstream, doctors, parents, athletes and coaches could acquire a greater understanding of them. Use could be made safer, clinical trials could be performed and dangerous overuse curbed.

The technology exists to test for levels of most of the substances on the "banned drugs" lists. What if we declared that certain levels of them in the body were acceptable, while excessive amounts would result in penalties? Athletes could satisfy their drive to be faster and stronger. Drugs could move from the black market to the legitimate sports-medicine community. Athletes could stop experimenting on themselves. It would be safer to take the substances, and with medical monitoring, there would be fewer negative side effects. . . . Track [performance] gets faster, nutrition gets more specific and training techniques improve.

Kate Schmidt, "Just Say Yes to Steroids—Learn, Make Better Choices," *Nicholls Worth*, October 18, 2007. http://thenichollsworth.com.

critics believe if sales were totally unregulated, the problem would certainly be much worse. Laws that require a valid prescription for steroid possession and use help limit the number of individuals who might end up abusing the drugs.

Protecting Young People from PED Abuse

Perhaps the most important function of laws against PEDs is to protect young people. Experts note that children and teenagers try to emulate the high-profile star athletes they see every day on TV and video clips. Many pro athletes today have muscular physiques like comic book superheroes, and young people may be drawn to take PEDs in hopes of looking the same. A 2014 survey by the Partnership for Drug-Free Kids found that the reported use of HGH among teens had doubled within a year. The rise in use among African American and Hispanic teens was even more pronounced. As Josie Feliz notes on the group's website, "These

Legalizing PEDs Would Not Lead to Safer Usage

Arguments that PEDs should be legal as long as their use is supervised by a doctor ignore the likely consequences. April Ashby of the Marquette University Law School says legalizing PEDs would be a slippery slope to further abuse.

> Doping threatens the health of athletes. . . . Legalizing steroid use would not solve these problems. The side effects listed in the National Center for Biotechnology Information (a part of the National Institute [*sic*] of Health) article are not restricted to improper use of steroids. . . .
>
> Law students, and indeed lawyers, are fond of the slippery slope argument. I think it finds a comfortable place in this debate. It's a slippery slope between allowing steroid use with proper medical supervision and eliminating anti-doping regulations. Where is the line to be drawn? Will it now be illegal to use steroids only if taken without proper medical supervision? How can proper medical supervision be proven? How does an athlete prove that the steroids in his or her body were as a result of proper medical supervision and not other means? What about athletes who use more than the recommended dose? . . . It's difficult to see how regulating the use of steroids in sports is workable.

April Ashby, "Why Steroids Have No Place in Sports," *Marquette University Law School Faculty Blog*, October 20, 2010. http://law.marquette.edu.

VIEWPOINT

findings underscore teens' growing interest in performance enhancing substances, as well as the need for tighter regulation and more accurate labeling of 'fitness-enhancing' over-the-counter products."[23]

Teens, both male and female, may feel pressured toward self-improvement and be vulnerable to aggressive product promotions that promise gains in muscle mass, improved athletic performance, and enhanced appearance. Typical is the story of a high-school wrestler in Iowa. Finding that steroids were easy to get at his local gym, he bought a bottle of testosterone and a syringe to improve his performance during wrestling season. He began injecting the drug at home, but ignored advice to use a different needle each time. Instead he would heat the needle over a flame in hopes of sterilizing it. One day at wrestling practice, the swollen injection area on his shoulder started to feel hot and very painful. The boy's coach sent him to the hospital with a serious infection. When the boy admitted to using steroids, he was suspended from school for a week and thrown off the wrestling team. He was fortunate not to face legal or medical troubles for his usage.

> "These findings [of increasing use] underscore teens' growing interest in performance enhancing substances, as well as the need for tighter regulation and more accurate labeling of 'fitness-enhancing' over-the-counter products."[23]
>
> —Josie Feliz, representative for the Partnership for Drug-Free Kids.

Were PED laws to disappear, the number of children and teens who turn to anabolic steroids and other performance-enhancing drugs would likely be much larger. "Amateur athletes, including high school and perhaps younger participants, look to their heroes for examples of how to succeed in sport," says Thomas H. Murray, president emeritus of the Hastings Center, a nonprofit bioethics research institute. "If doping was allowed, we could expect non-elite athletes to pursue the latest advances in performance enhancing drugs just as they buy the latest running shoes, bikes, or tennis rackets."[24]

Safe When Taken Under Doctor's Supervision

Some observers argue that PEDs, for all their health risks, offer tremendous benefits in strength, endurance, and healing ability

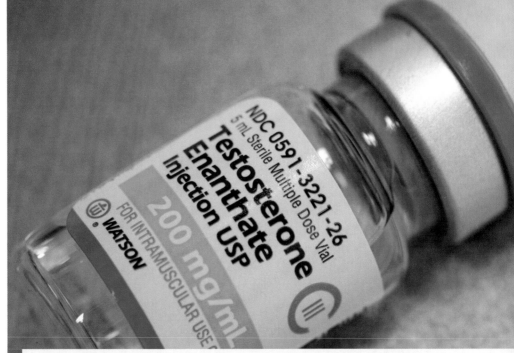

Injecting PEDs such as testosterone poses a risk of infection from improperly sterilized needles. Some advocates argue that making PEDs legal would reduce this risk because users would be monitored by a doctor.

to elite athletes and amateurs alike. These people insist that possessing and using PEDs should be legal for a number of reasons. The main reason for legalizing PEDs is to ensure that their use is monitored by a doctor. Advocates argue that this would make athletes much safer. Anabolic steroids are already prescribed to certain patients to help them gain weight, develop muscle mass, and treat certain kinds of anemia. Supporters believe this policy should be extended to athletes who wish to use PEDs to improve their performance. Under a doctor's supervision, users can be guided to take the safe dosage of a drug and to cycle off the drug when necessary. "The biggest problem with AS [anabolic steroids] is that they are obtained illegally, and then self-administered in secret by athletes who are not trained to identify overuse or to scale their dose appropriately," according to Bennett Foddy and Julian Savulescu, professors of science and ethics at Oxford University. "Like many behind-the-counter drugs, steroids can be taken safely but it is not safe enough to take them on your own. It would be much safer to take steroids for performance enhancement if they could be administered and monitored by a doctor. Such sports doctors could be held responsible for their athlete's health."[25] Moreover, if PEDs were legal, the efforts to make the drugs un-detectable by tests would no longer be necessary. Some argue that emphasis in manufacturing PEDs would entirely be placed on making the drugs safer and more effective.

New Opportunities for Research and Testing

Some medical experts see another benefit of legalizing PEDs: more extensive studies of the drugs. As it stands, there have been few studies of the long-term effects of PEDs such as ana-bolic steroids because usage is not only considered dangerous but is also illegal. Doctors can prescribe anabolic steroids only to treat certain specific conditions. As a result, what is known about the drugs' effect on athletes and other users is mostly limited to doctors' observations and the users' own accounts.

How to go about studying PED abuse has always been con-troversial. As the Mayo Clinic states on its website, "It is impos-sible for researchers to design studies that would accurately test the effects of large doses of steroids on athletes, because giving participants such high doses would be unethical. This means that the effects of taking anabolic steroids at very high doses haven't been well-studied."[26] Whereas legalizing anabolic steroids would not change the ethical problems with high-dosage tests, it would at least allow carefully controlled studies of steroid use, some-thing that has been done only rarely and with limited resources. Also, legalization would enable researchers to test each of the so-called designer drugs that regularly appear. These are exotic new PEDs, from hormone supplements to stimulants, that are designed to evade testing and that have had no approved medi-cal use other than as a performance enhancer. Such studies, ex-perts believe, would offer great benefits to the health and safety of athletes and other users of PEDs.

An Enormous Waste of Time and Money

A growing number of critics think laws against PEDs are a waste of the government's time, energy, and money. They insist that laws have no hope of holding back the tide of increasing PED use among athletes and the general public. When the financial rewards of playing Major League Baseball or NFL football are so great (the average MLB player makes more than $4 million per year) players are willing to risk fines, suspensions, and even jail time in order to get a competitive edge with anabolic steroids, HGH, or other PEDs. Revelations of steroid use have become so common that the public no longer seems to care. In the entertainment world, an increasing number of movie stars and rappers look like comic book superheroes with their PED-aided physiques and six-pack abs. As for amateur bodybuilders or weekend warriors, they see PED use all around them and come to feel that doping is a valid option. Some experts also believe the PED laws are basically interfering with people's right to improve themselves. Dr. Charles Yesalis says, "When I think of these laws, well, that would be like arresting and prosecuting a movie actress for some type of cosmetic surgery because she is not what you think."[27] And finally, there is the question of expense. Governments and sports organizations spend millions on investigations and tests, while elite athletes and their doctors either develop ways to mask their PED use or move on to newer, more exotic versions. The few offenders that are caught, critics say, are not worth the expense.

> "When I think of these laws [against PEDs], well, that would be like arresting and prosecuting a movie actress for some type of cosmetic surgery because she is not what you think."[27]
>
> —Dr. Charles Yesalis, professor of health policy and sport science at Penn State University.

An Unlikely Prospect

No matter the number of arrests made, it is unlikely that federal and state laws against PEDs will be scrapped anytime soon. Medical experts continue to emphasize the dangers of doping and particularly the risk to young people. Despite some practical benefits to legalization, most people believe professional and amateur sports should be drug free, and PEDs should continue to be regulated under the law.

In January 2013 American cyclist Lance Armstrong admitted to talk-show host Oprah Winfrey that he had used illegal doping to win his record-breaking seven titles at the Tour de France, cycling's most prestigious and grueling event. Armstrong, a cancer survivor from Austin, Texas, brought new attention to the sport of cycling, particularly in the United States, with his streak of dramatic wins. Then in October 2012 the Union Cycliste Internationale, cycling's main governing body, stripped Armstrong of his seven titles and banned him for life, citing growing evidence of his having used blood-doping drugs like EPO that boost endurance.

For a decade Armstrong had denied using illegal drugs during his victories. He had attacked his accusers, some of whom were former teammates, as liars and publicity seekers. In his interview with Winfrey, however, Armstrong conceded that his cycling career had been a big lie. With little show of emotion, he admitted that he was a ruthless competitor who needed to win at all costs. Armstrong went on to say that at the time he did not view his behavior as cheating. "I looked up the definition of cheat, and it is to gain an advantage over a rival or foe, and I didn't view [doping] that way," he said. "I viewed it as a level playing field."[28] He assumed that other top riders were doing the same thing he did. He also contended that winning such an arduous three-week race was almost impossible without the help of PEDs. Indeed, Armstrong is not the only recent Tour de France winner to be stripped of the title for doping. American Floyd Landis won the 2006 race but was later disqualified for a failed drug test. In 2012 Spaniard Alberto Contador was stripped of his 2010 title after a prolonged investigation turned up evidence of doping.

Loss of the Public's Confidence

The scandals involving Armstrong, Landis, and Contador caused some fans of professional cycling to abandon the sport. Many who continue to attend the race stages or watch on TV still regard any breakthrough performance with suspicion. In the 2015 Tour de France, British cyclist Chris Froome left all his rivals behind on the first mountain stage of the race, a brutal climb to the summit of La Pierre-Saint-Martin. Froome, who eventually won the 2015 race, drew questions from journalists and longtime fans about possible doping. Supporters urged Froome and his coaches on Team Sky to silence the critics by releasing the detailed data gathered that day about his performance and physical condition. Team Sky refused on the grounds that sharing the data would reveal too much about Froome's training methods and strategy to other teams and riders. After days of controversy Team Sky finally released a portion of Froome's data. However, some observers saw this move as a bad precedent. "From here, any professional cyclist who puts in a surprise performance might now have to face similar requests for their numbers and other private information to be released in order to be hauled over the coals in the court of public opinion,"[29] says cycling expert Craig Fry.

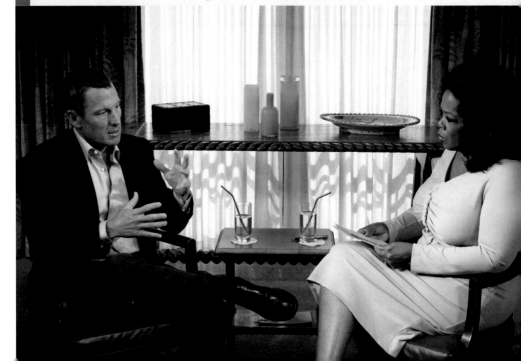

After more than a decade of denials, cyclist Lance Armstrong admitted to talk-show host Oprah Winfrey that he had indeed used PEDs to help him win the Tour de France seven consecutive times, although he also said he did not view their use as cheating. As a result of the scandal, Armstrong was banned from the sport for life.

The episode with Froome shows how atypical sports achievements immediately fall under suspicion. It also illustrates the extent to which athletes now have to go to convince the press and the public that they are clean, that they do not need PEDs to succeed. After a string of PED-related scandals in several sports, cynical fans have come to suspect that record-breaking performances are probably achieved by doping.

PEDs as a Form of Cheating

For many sports fans PED use raises a question of fairness. They see the use of PEDs as a form of cheating. They believe an athlete should rely on his or her own natural talent and ability, not on drugs and chemicals. Since cheating is not allowed in sports and games—a rule that goes back to the schoolyard—fans argue that PEDs should be illegal, and users should be punished or banned. In other words, most fans want a so-called level playing field in which no competitor has an unfair advantage of any kind. And using PEDs strikes many fans as the ultimate example of an unfair advantage.

A large number of athletes agree that peers who use PEDs are cheaters and should suffer the consequences. Greg LeMond, the only American cyclist to have won the Tour de France before Lance Armstrong, knows firsthand how much hard work it takes to succeed in professional cycling, and he disdains modern cyclists who resort to cheating with PEDs. LeMond cast doubt on Armstrong's success long before Armstrong admitted to doping. LeMond had learned from his former bike crew about Armstrong's shady practices—the syringes, IVs, bags of blood. Convinced that Armstrong was doping, LeMond finally told an interviewer in 2001, "If Lance is clean, it is the greatest comeback in the history of sports. If he isn't, it would be the greatest fraud."[30] For several years afterward, LeMond was practically ostracized from the sport for his comments. When Armstrong confessed and LeMond was proven correct, he claimed to have no sympathy for

> "If Lance is clean, it is the greatest comeback in the history of sports. If he isn't, it would be the greatest fraud."[30]
>
> —Greg LeMond, American cyclist and three-time champion of the Tour de France.

46

Armstrong. LeMond believes that stripping Armstrong of his titles was the only proper response to such blatant cheating.

Whereas many athletes like LeMond view doping as cheating, relatively few speak out on the subject. One notable exception is former New York Yankee Reggie Jackson, one of baseball's top-ten all-time sluggers. "You can't be breaking records hitting 200 home runs in three or four seasons. The greatest hitters in the history of the game didn't do that,"[31] Jackson remarked in 2004 about the state of modern MLB power-hitting. Jackson, whose career ended just as the steroid era in baseball was beginning, has been outspoken in his belief that players who pumped up their home run statistics with steroids have no place in baseball's Hall of Fame.

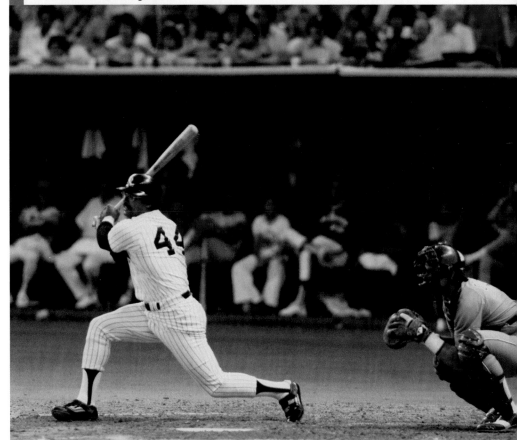

Baseball Hall of Famer Reggie Jackson, who retired from the sport after the 1987 season, is one of the few athletes who have publicly expressed disapproval of PED use. The reputation of Major League Baseball was badly tarnished after it was revealed that players who were shattering longstanding batting records beginning in 1998 had been using PEDs.

PED Users Don't Belong in Baseball's Hall of Fame

Cheating by using PEDs to get a competitive edge should not be rewarded. It is unfair to those who play fair, and it sends the wrong message to young fans. These are the views of Jim Bunning, US senator and former major league pitcher, who was elected to baseball's Hall of Fame in 1996.

The Hall of Fame is filled with baseball greats who set their records through nothing more than a lot of blood, sweat, and tears. They worked hard to get where they are today and if you want to know how they feel about sharing the stage with players who took shortcuts to beat their records, just go to the Hall of Fame dinner on Sunday night. The message is simple—cheaters need not apply. . . .

Whether major league players like it or not, they serve as role models to our nation's youth, who look up to them and want to one day be like them. If players who cheat to gain entrance into baseball's most elite club are given a free pass, it sends a terrible message to our nation's young athletes that it is OK to cheat. I don't think that's right. When I was a kid, I was taught that if you really wanted something in life you had to work hard to get it. There are no shortcuts in life.

Jim Bunning, "Steroid Users Have No Place in Hall of Fame," *US News & World Report*, July 21, 2009. www.usnews.com.

The Attraction of PED-Aided Performances

Professional sports leagues and the media can be cynical in the way they exploit the performances of athletes on PEDs. One of the most famous episodes was the 1998 National League home run chase. At the time the most famous record in American pro sports was the single season home run record of 61, set by the Yankees' Roger Maris in 1961. Maris's record, surpassing Babe Ruth's hallowed total of 60, had endured for thirty-seven years when the St. Louis Cardinals' Mark McGwire and the Chicago Cubs' Sammy Sosa suddenly began slamming round-trippers at a prodigious rate during the 1998 season. As the heavily muscled players approached Maris's record, people who ordinarily had no interest in baseball started checking the sports page or TV sports reports for the latest news about the home run derby. Reporters swarmed the stars for interviews after each game. Little attention was paid to the bottle of androstenedione, a steroid precursor, spotted in McGwire's locker one night in August. On September

Baseball's Hall of Fame Should Include Steroid Users

Keeping great baseball players out of the Hall of Fame simply because they used steroids is a mistake. Sportswriter Ted Berg argues that steroids were not banned when players used them in the 1990s and the past can't be changed.

> Some voters have said, quite reasonably, that they will vote for players from baseball's so-called Steroid Era but not those who have been found guilty of cheating. . . . But then, there's almost no doubt some players who were never caught cheating did indeed cheat. And if one of those guys earns a plaque, it hardly seems fair to deny the honor to players who confessed their guilt. . . .

> What happened happened. Until 2003, Major League Baseball and its teams did nothing to prevent players from taking anabolic steroids to enhance their performances, and so many players did. It's unfortunate, but it really shouldn't diminish the on-field accomplishments of that era. . . .

> Including a character clause in the voting criteria puts many baseball writers in the impossible position of retroactively policing men they never knew for taking actions no one tried to stop. It's time to take morality out of the picture and put great baseball players in the Hall of Fame.

Ted Berg, "4 Reasons the Baseball Hall of Fame Should Include Steroids Users," *USA Today*, December 27, 2013. http://ftw.usatoday.com.

8, fans across the nation cheered as McGwire hit his 62nd homer of the year, with nearly a month to go in the season. The pair went back and forth in their competition until McGwire finished the season with an astonishing total of 70 home runs to Sosa's 66. In a sport where records are usually broken by tiny increments, the two sluggers had left the old home run mark far behind. Interest in baseball had reached its highest point in years, and team owners were thrilled.

Soon, however, stories began to circulate about PED use and players "juicing" to increase their strength. The San Francisco Giants' Barry Bonds, a formerly slender superstar who had bulked up suspiciously, surpassed McGwire with a total of 73 homers in 2001. Six years later, Bonds also broke Hank Aaron's career home run record. By then fans realized that something was wrong, that balls were flying out of the park at ridiculous rates. Slugger Jose Canseco admitted to juicing and revealed that use of anabolic steroids was rife in the sport. The baseball record book, with its numbers that were familiar to every longtime fan, had been rewritten—some would say ruined—by cheaters. Philip Hersh, a sportswriter for the *Chicago Tribune*, says fans should have known it was too good to be true. "The Sosa-McGwire home run derby was indeed a fraud," says Hersh, "but it had become too much fun to ignore with a cynical, knowing shrug."[32] Todd McFarlane, a wealthy fan who paid $10 million for some of McGwire's home run balls, remains sad and disillusioned by the whole affair. "The reason it's still a dagger in the heart," says McFarlane, "is because we fell in love. We wanted it to be romantic and pure and innocent and fun, but it wasn't."[33]

> "The Sosa-McGwire home run derby was indeed a fraud, but it had become too much fun to ignore with a cynical, knowing shrug."[32]
>
> —*Chicago Tribune* sportswriter Philip Hersh.

Critics of what has become known as the steroid era in baseball say team owners and league officials had to know that players were using PEDs, but they conveniently looked the other way because the results were so profitable. "Baseball players before 2003 had nothing to fear from regulation or league policing, since there was absolutely no testing in place," says sports journalist

Christopher Hayes. "It was impossible to get caught, and the league sent the message from the very top that it would not only countenance but greatly reward those who cheated."[34] Owners have always denied knowledge of PED use at the time. However, according to Canseco, "They knew what I was doing. They knew what the other baseball players were doing, if they were involved in taking steroids. Owners knew it. Players Association knew it."[35] In any case, as public outrage grew in the 2000s, owners joined with the players union to finally set up a mandatory testing program for testosterone supplements and other PEDs. In the last five years only one player has topped even 50 home runs in a season.

Letting Athletes Maximize Their Ability

Some observers think tougher rules on PEDs merely prevent athletes from reaching their potential. A large part of pro sports' appeal, they say, is watching talented individuals perform at their absolute peak level. Fans attend games or watch broadcasts hoping to witness something they have never seen before—a mammoth home run, an acrobatic dunk, a burst of blazing speed to reach the end zone. PEDs enable athletes to develop strength, speed, and endurance beyond what was once thought possible. They open new horizons for athletic achievement. Some argue the best policy—and the one that would be most fair—is to legalize PEDs for all competitors. For example, sports business expert Chris Smith insists that doping is just another way athletes train to perform at that peak level. He believes that, given the chance, most athletes would use drugs to achieve better performances and that allowing all players to use PEDs would just create a different kind of fairness:

> Not only would the playing field suddenly be even for all players, it would be at a higher level. A huge part of watching sports is witnessing the very peak of human athletic ability, and legalizing performance enhancing drugs would help athletes climb even higher. Steroids and doping will help pitchers to throw harder, home runs to go further, cyclists to charge for longer and sprinters to test the very limits of human speed.[36]

Like Smith, advocates of blanket legalization also point out that athletes rise above their competitors for many reasons. Using PEDs would only be one more tool in developing their abilities.

> "Balco was exposed and the chemist went to prison. Is this evidence that doping control can work effectively? Or does it show that ultimately the effort will be futile because other chemists, other labs, and more willing athletes will inevitably pop up?"[38]
>
> —Thomas H. Murray, former president of the Hastings Center, a research institute dedicated to bioethics.

If PEDs were available to all pro athletes, the top performers would still be those who train harder, practice more, exhibit more discipline, and avoid mistakes on the field or court. Critics of current drug policies often observe that steroids could not improve Barry Bonds's extraordinary hand-eye coordination or propel his bat at the perfect angle to send a baseball over the fence. The benefits that athletes get from taking PEDs cannot give them natural ability or replace the hard work they do to develop their craft. Legalized PEDs, including steroids, HGH, EPO, and stimulants, would simply allow athletes in all sports to maximize their physical capabilities. Instead of being one-sided or unfair, competition would be more intense than ever. And this would be exciting and highly entertaining for sports fans.

Norman Fost, director of the Medical Ethics Program at the University of Wisconsin, believes that, in the interest of fair competition, all athletes should have access to PEDs if they want them. Fost admits that he dislikes the use of PEDs and would never use them himself. Yet he also flatly declares, "There is no coherent argument to support the view that enhancing performance is unfair; if it were, we would ban coaching and training. Competition can be unfair if there is unequal access to particular enhancements, but equal access can be achieved more predictably by deregulation than by prohibition."[37]

Easing the Difficulty of Policing Sports

Some argue that legalizing PEDs would actually promote fairness by setting simpler rules. As things stand, professional sports leagues and international sports bodies have a bewildering tangle

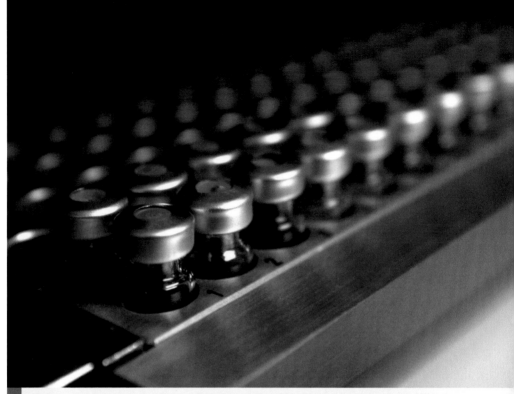

Vials containing urine samples await testing at the UCLA Olympic Analytical Laboratory. Tetrahydrogestrinone (THG) is a synthetic anabolic steroid that was designed to evade tests intended to detect traces of PEDs in a person's urine.

of rules and regulations about PED use and testing. They spend enormous sums trying to catch offenders, and doping athletes go to great lengths to avoid getting caught. In the end athletes with medical advisers who can help them mask their drug use evade the rules, while users who are less sophisticated or lack the same connections suffer the penalties.

Thomas H. Murray, former president of the Hastings Center, a research institute dedicated to bioethics, points to the BALCO scandal as an example:

The synthetic anabolic steroid tetrahydrogestrinone (THG)—now infamous as "the clear" peddled by the Balco lab—was created by an independent chemist. Its selling point was that the processes by which samples were prepared for testing by the anti-doping labs made the drug undetectable. The lab got its hands on a sample of THG, deciphered its chemistry, and adapted their procedures to detect it. Balco was exposed and the chemist went to prison. Is this evidence that doping control can work effectively? Or does it show that ultimately the effort will be futile because other chemists, other labs, and more willing athletes will inevitably pop up?"[38]

Allowing athletes to use PEDs openly would not only save sports organizations a great deal of time and money, some critics argue, but it would also end the disparity between those who get caught and those who do not. This would return the focus to which athlete has the better backhand or breaststroke, not to which can hire the best chemists.

Fairness Versus Freedom

Finally, some commentators look at PED use in light of personal freedom. They insist that each athlete should be free to pursue excellence however he or she chooses. What is truly unfair, they say, is trying to prevent athletes from improving themselves. The intrusive tests and constant surveillance to prevent drug use are heavy-handed attempts to enforce on athletes a dated morality. The methods required to enforce a ban on PEDs affect the freedom and dignity of athletes on a daily basis. Advocates for personal freedom maintain that questions of possible harm from PED use should be left to the individual and his or her advisers. They say that if society believes fairness means the right to make decisions about one's own body, this right must be extended to athletes, who depend on their physical condition for their livelihood.

How Effective Are Tests for Performance-Enhancing Drugs?

In 2013 researchers at the University of British Columbia (UBC) announced their development of a DNA test for blood doping. The new test examines athletes' blood for proteins to find if they have received a transfusion of another person's blood. It is designed to be cheaper, faster, and easier to administer than the previous version. Despite these claims and the fact that the USADA helped fund the research, other experts claim the new test is not very useful. It was originally supposed to be administered as a simple finger-prick test, one that could be used by volunteer doping control officers at the Olympics. However, the test does not work on such a small amount of blood, requiring instead a full tablespoon. The test also can be circumvented by various tricks that athletes and their handlers use, such as skimming away white blood cells—which can be detected as foreign—before transfusing the donor blood. In addition, the researchers at the University of British Columbia admit their test might lead to ethical concerns about privacy. "There may be a bit of a block to collecting athletes' genetic data,"[39] says James Rupert, associate professor in the School of Kinesiology at UBC. For now antidoping officials will probably stick with the current test. Christiane Ayotte, head of an antidoping lab in Montreal, Canada, says the current technique is well tested and accepted in court. "We already have the equipment, it has standing in courts and it's foolproof,"[40] says Ayotte.

> "We already have the equipment [for PED testing], it has standing in courts and it's foolproof."[40]
>
> —Christiane Ayotte, head of an antidoping lab in Montreal, Canada.

Difficulties of Detection

Blood doping, whether done by transfusion or by taking banned PEDs such as EPO or synthetic oxygen carriers, has been employed by athletes for decades. American Olympic sprinter Marion

Jones and boxer Shane Mosley are just two of the high-profile athletes who have been caught using EPO. Blood doping by transfusion has generally been more difficult to detect. An athlete can receive a transfusion of blood from someone of the same blood type or receive his or her own blood, which has been drawn at an earlier date and stored for later use. In fact, the current test for blood doping cannot detect autologous transfusions (i.e., transfusions of an athlete's own blood), the most prevalent form of blood doping. This is because the transfused blood is so similar to the old blood.

Blood doping works by boosting the oxygen-transporting capacity of an athlete's blood as it moves from the lungs to the muscles. During intense exercise, the body uses as much as twenty times more oxygen compared to when it is at rest. A sudden increase of hemoglobin, an oxygen-carrying protein inside red blood cells, raises an athlete's energy level and endurance. A test for so-called homologous transfusions, or those that use another person's blood, appeared only in 2004, following twenty years of trial and error. Yet scientists are still confounded by autologous blood transfusions. The WADA's current strategy is to use an electronic record called the Athlete Biological Passport. Although testing for markers of blood doping has been used by athletic associations since the 1980s, only in 2009 was the new biological record instituted. According to the WADA website, "The fundamental principle of the Athlete Biological Passport (ABP) is to monitor selected biological variables over time that indirectly reveal the effects of doping rather than attempting to detect the doping substance or method itself."[41] It remains to be seen how successful such an indirect method will be.

Even if testing improves, athletes and trainers continue to find ways to dope without getting caught. One major strategy is called microdosing. Elite track athletes are so close in physical skill that the difference between winning and losing can come

> "The fundamental principle of the Athlete Biological Passport (ABP) is to monitor selected biological variables over time that indirectly reveal the effects of doping rather than attempting to detect the doping substance or method itself."[41]
>
> —World Anti-Doping Agency website.

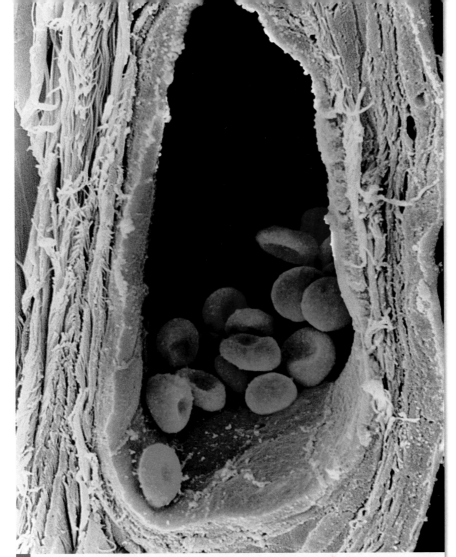

This image captured by a microscope shows red blood cells inside a vein. Because these cells carry oxygen, blood doping involves boosting their number in the bloodstream to increase the flow of oxygen from the lungs to the muscles, thereby increasing endurance.

down to marginal gains. These athletes can get the benefits they seek from very small amounts of steroids or EPO, and tiny concentrations of drugs can be very difficult to detect and measure. For example, testosterone taken in small amounts can evade the popular T/E ratio test, which compares the amount of testosterone to epitestosterone (a form of testosterone with the same type and number of atoms but in a different arrangement) in the body. Most individuals have a T/E ratio of 1 to 1, but since the ratio can be higher for many people, the WADA set the T/E ratio limit at 4 to 1. This gives athletes with ordinary ratios of T/E room to cheat. Adding to the testers' difficulties is the fact that the elevated T/E ratio quickly falls to normal for many people, just as the benefits of the drug are kicking in. Experts say this problem could be solved by adding tests for other markers of doping. However, issues of expense and privacy often intervene.

A Patchwork of Testing Procedures

In addition to concerns about the effectiveness of detection, the unevenness of testing procedures causes some officials and observers to worry that many athletes are not held to the same rigorous monitoring. Testing procedures vary widely from country to country and sport to sport. Officials must determine how many athletes to test and how they are chosen. During competition, athletes are chosen for testing based on rules set by each sport's

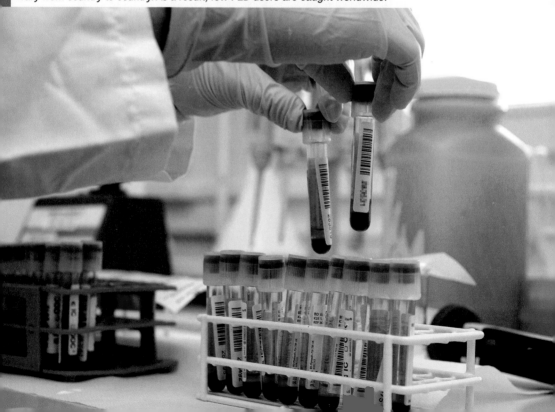

Although the World Anti-Doping Code establishes how antidoping programs, including blood testing, should be conducted, the reality is that competency and efficiency among drug testing labs (pictured) vary from country to country. As a result, few PED users are caught worldwide.

governing body. In track-and-field events, for example, the top three finishers plus a random selection of other competitors might be tested. In the off-season, the USADA requires all athletes to notify the group about their whereabouts so they can be located for out-of-competition testing. Athletes can be tested with the collection of blood or urine samples 365 days a year with no advance notice. The USADA also manages the results of the tests by informing athletes about the results and dealing with any potential violations of antidoping rules.

One reason why so few PED cheaters worldwide get caught is the large disparity among drug testing labs and their procedures. Problems of financing and oversight mean that some countries have limited staff and shoddy practices for testing. Although the WADA sets the World Anti-Doping Code, which describes how antidoping programs should be conducted by sports federations and national governments, too many countries lack the competence and efficiency necessary to meet these standards. Even supposedly tough measures like the so-called whereabouts requirements can be evaded. Athletes can miss three tests in twelve months before facing any sanction. The attempt to set up uniform standards and coordinate testing efforts is still new. For now the system remains just a global patchwork.

The Rationale for PED Testing

Despite these concerns, sports leagues and national sports bodies continue to pursue tougher testing programs for athletes. Their stated aim is to eliminate the use of PEDs in competitive athletics for reasons of health, safety, and fairness. But there is another motive that is just as urgent. As doping scandals have grabbed headlines in many sports, from Olympic track and field to professional cycling to Major League Baseball, officials have scrambled to bolster public confidence in their sports. At stake are millions of dollars in ticket sales, broadcasting rights, advertising, and sales of merchandise. Taking a strong stand on drug testing is seen as a way to uphold the integrity of a sport.

Yet professional leagues, Olympic committees, and groups like the WADA must deal with the hard reality of ruthless competition.

Athletes, coaches, and trainers will take great risks to get an edge and reach the top. As drug expert Jeannette Y. Wick explains,

> How much will they risk? *Sports Illustrated* interviewed a cohort of elite Olympic athletes, asking, "If you were given a performance-enhancing substance, you would not be caught, and you would win, would you take it?" Ninety-eight percent of athletes answered yes. When they changed the question to, "If you were given a performance-enhancing substance, and you would not be caught, win all competitions for 5 years, then die, would you take it?" More than 50% still said yes.[42]

Athletes themselves have millions at stake in the form of contracts and endorsements. If they are determined, they can find ways to foil tests for PEDs. "The ability to detect drug misuse is limited," says Wick. "Many athletes know the . . . pharmacology of the drugs they take better than a third-year pharmacy student does."[43] Thus PED testing is like a game of cops and robbers, with each side trying to outdo the other with cutting-edge chemistry and clever stratagems.

The Challenge of Testing for PEDs

With this in mind, designing adequate PED tests and testing procedures is a challenge. This is especially true regarding tests for anabolic steroids. The complex molecular chemistry of anabolic steroids makes them very difficult to detect in a sample of bodily fluids such as saliva, blood, or urine, and especially hard to distinguish from other substances. It is easier to test for exogenous anabolic steroids, which do not occur normally in the human body. Their presence in a test sample indicates that the subject is probably doping. However, testing for endogenous anabolic steroids, such as naturally occurring testosterone, is much trickier. The tester must determine whether the natural levels have been boosted artificially with pills or other aids. Normally the subject's T/E levels are compared to the statistical norm for males, but because natural variance occurs, some experts question the effectiveness of the T/E approach. Scientists have discussed replacing it with a carbon-isotope ratio test, a relatively simple method for comparing the ratios of carbon atoms in urine. In any case if the tests yield a positive result for PEDs, a confirmatory test is done to determine with a high degree of reliability whether the sample contains a banned substance.

Two factors that complicate such PED testing are false positives and false negatives. A false positive indicates a banned substance in a sample when none is present. A false negative is a failure to detect a banned substance that is present. Of the two, the false positive is much more serious. It can lead to an athlete being stripped of a gold medal or banned from competition despite the fact that no actual violation occurred. For example, a false positive may result from an athlete taking a prescription medicine that, unbeknownst to her or him, contains a banned substance. Sports organizations try to create special conditions for testing athletes with chronic or acute medical problems that require prescription drugs.

> "Many athletes know the . . . pharmacology of the drugs they take better than a third-year pharmacy student does."[43]
>
> —Drug expert Jeannette Y. Wick.

False positives due to prescription drugs can even cause problems for amateur athletes. In 2013 Texas-based amateur cyclist and triathlete Sloan Teeple was stunned to receive an eighteen-month ban from the USADA when he tested positive for a testosterone supplement, which he explained was prescribed by his doctor for a medical condition. The 44-year-old had applied for a waiver from USADA but was denied. "I was very up front with the racing community about my [testosterone] use," Teeple says. "I voluntarily told the [USADA] testers that I was using it when I was tested."[44] Amateur athletes like Teeple generally are tested only if they reach the upper echelons of their sport and are likely to finish near the top of the field.

As Teeple found, dealing with an accusation based on a false positive can be expensive and time consuming. Officials strive to virtually eliminate false positives, but this has proved difficult to

Testing for PEDs Is Accurate and Effective

Officials of the WADA believe their testing policies are extremely accurate and effective for catching cheaters who take PEDs. Dr. Gary Wadler, chairman of the WADA's Prohibited List and Methods Committee, explains why.

> The detection methods [of the WADA] are accurate and reliable. They undergo rigorous validation prior to being introduced. . . . WADA is, of course, keenly interested in the efficiency, as well as the effectiveness, of the global anti-doping system and supports research to help enhance testing efficiency. . . .
>
> Working collaboratively with national anti-doping agencies such as the US Anti-Doping Agency (USADA) in the sharing of information has uncovered the designer steroid THG, and WADA-certified laboratories continue to keep a watchful eye for previously unknown doping agents. . . .
>
> The [International Olympic Committee] retains ownership of the athlete's samples (blood and urine) for eight years following the Olympic Games. . . . During the ensuing eight years, if a technique is developed that would enable the detection of a prohibited substance . . . the stored specimen could be tested for that specific substance and the athlete would be held accountable.

Dr. Gary Wadler, "Dr. Gary Wadler of the World Anti-Doping Agency Gives His Answers to Your Questions (Part I)," *New York Times*, June 26, 2008. http://beijing2008.blogs.nytimes.com.

achieve. David E. Newton, an expert in chemistry and science education, explains the numbers:

> According to one fairly sophisticated mathematical analysis of this problem, the rate of false positives in sports antidoping programs can be expected to range from 0.0 percent to 0.53 percent. While that number does seem very low, one needs to remember the number of athletes tested each year, 146,539 in this particular study. In such a case, one might expect to find 777 false positives, a fairly large number.[45]

Testing at the Genetic Level

New evidence suggests that some of the world's athletes may be able to dope without fear of being detected at all. According to genetic researchers, some people have a gene that moderates T/E levels, keeping them low even if foreign steroids have

Testing for PEDs Will Never Catch All the Cheaters

Some believe antidoping tests will never be much more effective than they are today. Cheaters find too many ways to evade getting caught, say David Epstein, author of the book *The Sports Gene*, and Michael J. Joyner, physiologist at the Mayo Clinic in Rochester, Minnesota.

> As anti-doping authorities collect more biological passport data, they will have a better picture of what abnormal results look like, and can set the bar for a positive test less conservatively. And new biological markers that can be tested for evidence of doping will surely be discovered. But it is unlikely that anti-doping will reach the point where an athlete who is microdosing and carefully engineering their blood profile can't potentially slip through unnoticed. . . .
>
> Even as technology has improved, the proportion of worldwide samples that test positive remains at about 1 to 2 percent year after year. The dopers and anti-dopers may be in technological lockstep. . . .
>
> If you find the testing situation in Olympic sports depressing, remember that the WADA-approved testing regimen is the absolute gold standard in sports. Major League Baseball comes the closest—but not all that close—among the major pro sports leagues. The reason more athletes in those leagues aren't being sanctioned for doping probably isn't because it isn't occurring.

David Epstein and Michael J. Joyner, "Speed Bumps: Why It's So Hard to Catch Cheaters in Track and Field," Pro Publica, August 20, 2015. www.propublica.org.

VIEWPOINT

been introduced into the body. The frequency of this gene varies among different populations. Whereas only about 10 percent of Caucasians have it, it is found in about 30 to 40 percent of Japanese and Chinese. Athletes with this gene breeze through T/E ratio tests so that testers have no reason to follow up with another screening, such as a carbon isotope test, which might catch their doping.

> "If we really wanted to be technologically savvy about drug-testing, we'd have to have genetically personalized testing."[46]
>
> —David Epstein, an authority on genetics in sport.

To identify this gene, experts recommend adding genetic data to each athlete's Biological Passport, or personal database. "If we really wanted to be technologically savvy about drug-testing, we'd have to have genetically personalized testing,"[46] says David Epstein, an authority on genetics in sport. If the gene data revealed this specific gene in an athlete, then those individuals could be marked for more rigorous testing. People like Epstein believe that gathering genetic data might be the only way to catch cheaters who take advantage of their genetic makeup.

Nagging Questions About Testing

Questions about the effectiveness of PED testing refuse to go away, but so do claims that athletic associations may be ignoring or purposefully masking the results. The latest controversy involves a leaked database of twelve thousand blood tests of five thousand track athletes from 2001 to 2012. Analysis of the test results revealed that more than eight hundred of the athletes— about 16 percent of the total—had suspicious blood values that indicated doping. These athletes were highly successful in the years covered, winning roughly one-third of the medals awarded in endurance events in the Olympics and the International Association of Athletics Federations (IAAF) World Championships. The story set off shock waves in the track world, as gossip swirled about who was on the list. A few high-profile athletes like British runner Mo Farah, the defending Olympic champion in the 5,000- and 10,000-meter races, published their own blood results in an attempt to head off rumors. Such scandals reinforce the public

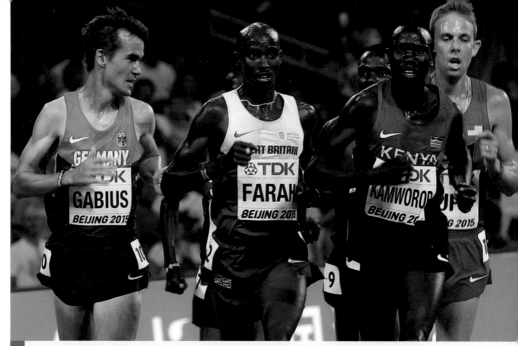

British runner Mo Farah took the unusual step of publishing his own blood test results to ward off rumors in the wake of a scandal stemming from the leak of a database containing a decade's worth of track-and-field athletes' test results—many of which were suspicious. Such scandals fuel public perception that PED testing is inadequate and a low priority for many sports organizations.

perception that tests for PEDs are inadequate at best and that sports organizations try to hide from their fans the reality about doping. Allegations that Russian athletes received banned substances from their government and conspired with doping control officers to falsify drug tests only add to the general cynicism.

Stories about doping athletes and failed drug tests seem to arise every few weeks. Organizations such as the WADA and the professional sports leagues in the United States continue to work at developing antidoping policies and testing procedures to keep their sports drug free. At the same time, there are plenty of athletes and trainers just as dedicated to eluding the tests and gaining the benefits of PEDs. This uneasy standoff seems unlikely to change for the foreseeable future.

Introduction: A Secret Doping Program

1. Quoted in Matthew Futterman, Sara Germano, and Paul Sonne, "Anti-Doping Commission Finds Russia Engaged in State-Sponsored Doping," *Wall Street Journal*, November 9, 2015. www.wsj.com.
2. Quoted in Futterman, Germano, and Sonne, "Anti-Doping Commission Finds Russia Engaged in State-Sponsored Doping."
3. Craig Calcaterra, "Fans Care About PEDs—Sometimes," NBC Sports, June 6, 2013. http://mlb.nbcsports.com.

Chapter 1: What Are the Facts?

4. Sean Gregory, "The Stream Is Over: A-Rod Admits to Manipulating Drug Tests," *Time*, November 5, 2014. http://time.com.
5. Quoted in Alexandra Pannoni, "Doping Rises Among High Schoolers, but Few Districts Test," *U.S. News & World Report*, August 11, 2014. www.usnews.com.
6. Quoted in Ryan Szivos, "Probing Question: Can Steroids Enhance Athletic Performance?," *Penn State News*, July 3, 2006. http://news.psu.edu.
7. Quoted in Barry Petchesky, "Why Don't We Let Injured Athletes Use PEDs?," *Deadspin* (blog), June 13, 2013. http://deadspin.com.
8. Quoted in Brittany Risher, "Creatine: What It Is, What It Does, and Its Side Effects," *Men's Health*, September 2, 2013. www.menshealth.com.

Chapter 2: How Dangerous Is the Use of Performance-Enhancing Drugs?

9. Quoted in Chris Colucci, "Big Dead Bodybuilders: The Ultimate Price of Pro Bodybuilding?," T Nation, April 30, 2015. www.t-nation.com.
10. MuscleK, "Update: Mike Matarazzo Is Dead but Blamed Steroids While Alive!," *Steroid Analysis* (blog), August 18, 2014. http://steroidanalysis.com.

11. Quoted in Ted Thornhill, "Fitness-Obsessed Bodybuilder Who Said He Was Invincible Died from 'Massive' Steroid Use After He Started Working Out Again Despite TWO Heart Attacks and THREE Strokes," *Daily Mail* (London), April 2, 2014. www.dailymail.co.uk.
12. Quoted in Lucy Carroll, "Young Men Dying from Heart Disease Linked to Steroid Use," *Sydney (Australia) Morning Herald*, February 27, 2014. www.smh.com.au.
13. Quoted in Miranda Hitti, "Pro Wrestler's Alleged Murder-Suicide Spurs Questions About Roid Rage and Anabolic Steroids," WebMD, June 27, 2007. www.webmd.com.
14. Quoted in Shirley S. Wang, "Scientists Warn of Risks from Growth Hormone," *Wall Street Journal*, March 24, 2014. www.wsj.com.
15. A. Marc Gillinov, "Performance-Enhancing Drugs in the Media Again," *Huffington Post*, January 16, 2014. www.huffington post.com.
16. Quoted in Carl T. Hall, "Steroids, Though Dangerous, Do Have Redeeming Qualities," SFGate, December 27, 2004. www.sf gate.com.
17. Quoted in Chris DiEugenio, "Playing with Steroids: A Chat with Dr. Charles Yesalis," T Nation, November 12, 2007. www.t-nation.com.
18. Quoted in Conal Andrews, "Former Team Doctor Claims EPO Is Not Harmful," Velonation, May 10, 2010. www.velonation .com.

Chapter 3: Should Performance-Enhancing Drugs Be Illegal?

19. Quoted in Chuck Penfold, "Germany's Anti-doping Law Comes into Force," Deutsche Welle, December 18, 2015. www.dw.com.
20. Dr. Thomas Bach, "Bach: PED Testing Not an Expense, but an Investment in Future of Athletics," *Sport Digest*, November 15, 2013. http://thesportdigest.com.
21. Quoted in Mark Lamport-Stokes, "World Anti-Doping Agency Calls for Closer Collaboration in War on Drugs," Reuters, December 28, 2015. www.reuters.com.

22. Harrison G. Pope Jr. et al., "Adverse Health Consequences of Performance-Enhancing Drugs: An Endocrine Society Scientific Statement," *Endocrine Reviews*, December 17, 2013. www.ncbi.nlm.nih.gov.

23. Josie Feliz, "National Study: Teens Report Higher Use of Performance Enhancing Substances," Partnership for Drug-Free Kids, July 22, 2014. www.drugfree.org.

24. Thomas Murray, "Debate: Should Performance-Enhancing Drugs Be Legalized?," *Blue Ridge Outdoors*, October 17, 2013. www.blueridgeoutdoors.com.

25. Quoted in David E. Newton, *Steroids and Doping in Sports.* Santa Barbara, CA: ABC-CLIO, 2014, p. 124.

26. Mayo Clinic, "Performance-Enhancing Drugs: Know the Risks," Mayo Clinic. www.mayoclinic.org.

27. Quoted in Jack Moore, "Germany's Absurd New PED Law and Why It Won't Fix Anything," Vice Sports, December 1, 2014. https://sports.vice.com.

Chapter 4: Do Performance-Enhancing Drugs Undermine Fairness in Sports?

28. Quoted in Aaron Hersh, "Armstrong Doping Confession: Key Quotes," *Triathlete*, January 18, 2013. http://triathlon.competitor.com.

29. Craig Fry, "The Curious Case of Chris Froome: Why He and Cycling Deserve Better," Cycling Tips, July 23, 2015. http://cyclingtips.com.au.

30. Quoted in Matt Majendie, "Can the Lies and Bullying Be Forgiven?," CNN, August 20, 2014. http://edition.cnn.com.

31. Associated Press, "Slugger Doesn't Believe Today's Athletes," ESPN.com, March 17, 2004. http://espn.go.com.

32. Philip Hersh, "Sammy Sosa–Mark McGwire Home Run Chase? We Should Have Known Better," *Chicago Tribune*, October 12, 2015. http://my.chicagotribune.com.

33. Quoted in Greg Bishop, "After Drug Revelations, Redefining '98 Home Run Chase," *New York Times,* July 4, 2009. www.nytimes.com.

34. Christopher Hayes, "The Steroids Era Was Just Like the Housing Bubble: How MLB Incentivized Widespread Fraud," Deadspin, July 19, 2012. http://deadspin.com.

35. Quoted in Rebecca Leung, "MLB Swings Back at Steroid Claims," CBS News, February 15, 2005. www.cbs.news .com.

36. Chris Smith, "Why It's Time to Legalize Steroids in Professional Sports," *Forbes*, August 24, 2012. www.forbes.com.

37. Quoted in "Do Athletes Gain an Unfair Advantage by Using Performance Enhancing Drugs?," ProCon.org, December 12, 2008. http://sportsanddrugs.procon.org.

38. Thomas H. Murray, "Sports Enhancement," Hastings Center. www.thehastingscenter.org.

Chapter 5: How Effective Are Tests for Performance-Enhancing Drugs?

39. Quoted in Camille Bains, "UBC Researchers Develop DNA Test to Catch Doping Cheats in Elite Sports," *Globe and Mail* (Toronto), October 18, 2013. www.theglobeandmail.com.

40. Quoted in Bains, "UBC Researchers Develop DNA Test to Catch Doping Cheats in Elite Sports."

41. World Anti-Doping Agency, "Athlete Biological Passport." www.wada-ama.org.

42. Jeannette Y. Wick, "Performance-Enhancing Drugs: A New Reality in Sports?," *Pharmacy Times*, March 13, 2014. www .pharmacytimes.com.

43. Wick, "Performance-Enhancing Drugs."

44. Quoted in Frederick Dreier, "Doping Cops Take Aim at Amateur Athletes," *Wall Street Journal*, December 23, 2015. www .wsj.com.

45. Newton, *Steroids and Doping in Sports*, p. 84.

46. Quoted in Nick Harris, "Born to Cheat! How World Class Athletes Can Take Drugs . . . and Get Away With It," *Daily Mail* (London), August 24, 2013. www.dailymail.co.uk.

International Olympic Committee (IOC)
Chateau de Vidy
Case postale 356
1001 Lausanne, Switzerland
+41-21-621-61-11
www.olympic.org

The IOC is the supreme authority of the Olympic Movement and manages collaboration between all parties of the Olympic family, including national Olympic committees. It also oversees the drug policies related to Olympic competition.

National Collegiate Athletic Association (NCAA)
700 W. Washington St.
PO Box 6222
Indianapolis, IN 46206
(317) 917-6222
www.ncaa.org

The NCAA is an organization devoted to safeguarding the well-being of student-athletes and equipping them to succeed on the playing field and in the classroom. The NCAA includes a Sports Science Institute, which promotes safety and wellness for college student-athletes and develops guidelines for antidoping and substance abuse policies.

National Strength and Conditioning Association (NSCA)
1885 Bob Johnson Dr.
Colorado Springs, CO 80906
(800) 815-6826
www.nsca.com

The NSCA supports and disseminates research-based knowledge and its practical application to improve performance and fitness. This includes current information and statistics about performance-enhancing drugs and their relation to strength training and conditioning.

Taylor Hooton Foundation (THF)

PO Box 2104
Frisco, TX 75034
(972) 403-7300
http://taylorhooton.org

The THF is a nonprofit organization dedicated to educating youth and their adult influencers about the dangers of appearance and performance enhancing drugs, including anabolic steroids, HGH, and unregulated dietary supplements.

US Anti-Doping Agency (USADA)

5555 Tech Center Dr., Suite 200
Colorado Springs, CO 80919
(719) 785-2000
www.usada.org

The USADA is the national antidoping organization in the United States for Olympic and Paralympic competition. The organization manages in-competition and out-of-competition testing, results management processes, drug reference resources, and athlete education about PEDs.

US Food and Drug Administration (FDA)

10903 New Hampshire Ave.
Silver Spring, MD 20993
(888) 463-6332
www.fda.gov

The FDA is responsible for protecting the public health by assuring the safety, effectiveness, and security of drugs, biological products, medical devices, the nation's food supply, cosmetics, and products that emit radiation. Among the drugs it regulates are PEDs of various kinds, including anabolic steroids.

World Anti-Doping Agency (WADA)

Stock Exchange Tower
800 Place Victoria (Suite 1700)

PO Box 120
Montreal, QC H4Z1B7
Canada
(514) 904-9232
www.wada-ama.org

The WADA monitors and aims to bring consistency to antidoping policies and regulations within sports organizations and governments worldwide. It oversees compliance with antidoping policies and coordinates antidoping efforts globally.

Books

Reed Albergotti, *Wheelmen: Lance Armstrong, the Tour de France, and the Greatest Sports Conspiracy Ever.* New York: Dutton, 2014.

Paul Anthony, *Sex and Sport and Drugs and Cheating: A Brief History of Sport and Cheating.* Nottingham, UK: DB, 2014.

Tim Elfrink and Gus Garcia-Roberts, *Blood Sport: Alex Rodriguez, Biogenesis, and the Quest to End Baseball's Steroid Era.* New York: Dutton, 2014.

David E. Newton, *Steroids and Doping in Sports.* Santa Barbara, CA: ABC-CLIO, 2014.

Andrew Tilin, *The Doper Next Door: My Strange and Scandalous Year on Performance-Enhancing Drugs.* Berkeley, CA: Counterpoint, 2011.

Internet Sources

David Epstein and Michael J. Joyner, "The Human Reasons Why Athletes Who Dope Get Away with It," Pro Publica, August 31, 2015. www.propublica.org/article/the-human-reasons-why-athletes-who-dope-get-away-with-it.

Amna Jamshad, "Performance Enhancing Drugs in the Olympic Games," *Premed Magazine*, April 1, 2014. www.premedmag.org/2014/04/01/performance-enhancing-drugs-in-the-olympic-games/.

Mark Lamport-Stokes, "World Anti-Doping Agency Calls for Closer Collaboration in War on Drugs," *Daily Mail* (London), December 28, 2015. http://www.dailymail.co.uk/wires/reuters/article-3376706/World-Anti-Doping-Agency-calls-closer-collaboration-war-drugs.html.

Alexandra Pannoni, "Doping Rises Among High Schoolers, but Few Districts Test," *U.S. News & World Report*, August 11, 2014. www.usnews.com/education/blogs/high-school-notes/2014/08/11/testing-high-school-athletes-for-doping-uncommon.

Chris Smith, "Why It's Time to Legalize Steroids in Professional Sports," *Forbes*, August 24, 2012. www.forbes.com/sites/chris smith/2012/08/24/why-its-time-to-legalize-steroids-in-profes sional-sports/#b2f5dc51c0db.

Websites

KidsHealth (http://kidshealth.org). A source of physician-reviewed information, KidsHealth provides a good overview of what steroids are and the dangers associated with their use.

LiveScience (www.livescience.com). This news and developments website includes a section titled "What Is Blood Doping?," which explains the science behind blood doping and how tests are designed to detect it.

The Mayo Clinic (www.mayoclinic.org). The Mayo Clinic is a non-profit worldwide leader in medical care, research, and education. Its website includes a section on PEDs, "Performance-Enhancing Drugs: Know the Risks."

National Institute on Drug Abuse (www.drugabuse.gov). This government organization is devoted to the prevention of drug abuse. The organization's website contains a section titled "Anabolic Steroid Abuse" that answers many frequently asked questions about the drugs and their risks.

Oregon Health and Science University (www.ohsu.edu). This website includes information about ATHENA (Athletes Targeting Healthy Exercise & Nutrition Alternatives) and ATLAS (Athletes Training & Learning to Avoid Steroids), two programs that address the dangers of PED use for female and male athletes, respectively.

INDEX

PICTURE CREDITS

ABOUT THE AUTHOR

John Allen is a writer living in Oklahoma City.